Get Started in Reflexology

In loving memory of my beloved mother

Daphne Marian Corner

Teach® Yourself

Get Started in Reflexology
Chris Stormer

For UK order enquiries: please contact Bookpoint Ltd,
130 Milton Park, Abingdon, Oxon OX14 4SB.
Telephone: +44 (0) 1235 827720. Fax: +44 (0) 1235 400454.
Lines are open 09.00–17.00, Monday to Saturday, with a 24-hour
message answering service. Details about our titles and how to
order are available at www.teachyourself.com

For USA order enquiries: please contact McGraw-Hill Customer
Services, PO Box 545, Blacklick, OH 43004-0545, USA.
Telephone: 1-800-722-4726. Fax: 1-614-755-5645.

For Canada order enquiries: please contact McGraw-Hill
Ryerson Ltd, 300 Water St, Whitby, Ontario L1N 9B6, Canada.
Telephone: 905 430 5000. Fax: 905 430 5020.

Long renowned as the authoritative source for self-guided
learning – with more than 50 million copies sold worldwide –
the **Teach Yourself** series includes over 500 titles in the fields of
languages, crafts, hobbies, business, computing and education.

British Library Cataloguing in Publication Data: a catalogue record
for this title is available from the British Library.

Library of Congress Catalog Card Number: on file.

First published in UK 1996 by Hodder Education, part of
Hachette UK, 338 Euston Road, London NW1 3BH.

First published in US 1996 by The McGraw-Hill Companies, Inc.

This edition published 2010.

Previously published as *Teach Yourself Reflexology.*

The **Teach Yourself** name is a registered trade mark of
Hodder Headline.

Typeset by MPS Limited, a Macmillan Company.

Printed in Great Britain for Hodder Education, an Hachette UK
Company, 338 Euston Road, London NW1 3BH, by CPI Cox &
Wyman, Reading, Berkshire RG1 8EX.

The publisher has used its best endeavours to ensure that the URLs
for external websites referred to in this book are correct and active
at the time of going to press. However, the publisher and the
author have no responsibility for the websites and can make no
guarantee that a site will remain live or that the content will remain
relevant, decent or appropriate.

Hachette UK's policy is to use papers that are natural, renewable
and recyclable products and made from wood grown in sustainable
forests. The logging and manufacturing processes are expected to
conform to the environmental regulations of the country of origin.

Impression number   10 9 8 7 6 5 4 3 2 1
Year   2014 2013 2012 2011 2010

Acknowledgements

To have Hodder Education as my publisher is indeed a privilege, as is the opportunity to re-edit and then rewrite this book, first published in 1996. I have come a long way since then and truly appreciate the opportunity to share this universal information far and wide.

My superb husband, John Fryer, is my 'rock'; always so supportive and encouraging. My two wonderful sons, Andrew and David, have long since left home, but continue to be 'there' for me. Meanwhile, my elderly Dad provides moral support, now that my beloved mother, Daphne Corner, has become an angel, constantly inspiring me from the other side.

I am eternally grateful to Sally Teixeira, Sarisha Harilal and Susanne Mason for stepping in at the last moment to help me out with the editing. Sally also assisted with changing the format of this publication; I am so grateful to you, Sally, for doing this; I could never have done it without you. Then there's Val Seddon, my 'Astral Mum', always imparting wonderful wisdom, as well as my dear friend, Kath Forster, who lovingly sends healing and support whenever required. At our divine Good Vibrations Health Sanctuary in Johannesburg is our amazing Sanctuary Angel, Leah Ramaliba, who constantly has a smile on her face and keeps things running smoothly while I travel the world presenting seminars and workshops.

There are literally thousands of reflexology students, teachers and practitioners worldwide, who have inspired me during the past 22 years, ever since I first became passionate about feet, along with a host of other natural healers, all of whom are very dear to me. Many, many thanks to you all! As for the numerous delegates who come to my seminars, it's their ongoing faith and encouragement that has kept me going for so long! I am in the fantastic position that I am in today because of them, so my heartfelt love and appreciation goes out to each and every one of them.

To you, dear reader, I honour your decision to take your understanding a step further, because without you, books like this would not be possible.

May you all enjoy abundant happiness and ultimate fulfilment every step of the way.

Contents

Meet the author

Having been in the medical world for ten years, I was a complete sceptic when first stumbling into reflexology in 1987. Even after qualifying, I wanted nothing to do with the feet! But a divorce left me with no means to bring up my two young sons and it was reflexology that stepped in and helped me out. Its popularity at our health studio led to the opening of the Reflexology Academy of Southern Africa in 1990, with international recognition following soon afterwards. Then in 1991, a presentation I gave on reflexology at an international congress in Beijing resulted in a stream of invitations to be a keynote speaker and also present full workshops and seminars worldwide. Since then, my feet have barely touched the ground. With such passion for feet, I am known throughout the world as the 'universal foot lady'!

Only got a minute?

Reflexology is an ancient art that brings together healing of the mind, body and soul, simply through the gentle massage of feet. Its effectiveness comes from knowing how perfectly feet reflect the physical body, in miniature, with each specific reflex point being linked to the corresponding part of the body.

By observing ongoing changes in the condition and appearance of feet, it is possible to gain further understanding of what is really going on at a much deeper level. This provides astonishing insight into how innermost thoughts and emotions can affect overall wellbeing; it also reveals the origins of the physical symptoms of distress and disease – where they come from.

Massaging feet should stimulate a healing response, mentally, physically, emotionally and spiritually, with the energy going to wherever it is needed. This brings everything back into perfect balance and puts things into perspective – particularly beneficial at times of confusion and chaos.

Fortunately everyone, no matter how young or old, can benefit from the wonders of reflexology, whether it is a one-off session or a series of treatments. Furthermore, it's an innate gift that everybody has from the time of being able to stand on their own two feet! All that's required to practise reflexology is the desire to take the next step towards better health and make a positive difference.

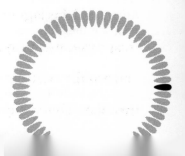

5 Only got five minutes?

Reflexology is an ancient healing art that has its roots in many different cultures throughout the world. It stems from an awareness of just how important feet are in healing the mind, body and spirit. This has been recognized from deepest Africa to the Far East, from the Americas to Europe and beyond.

Today, as one of the world's leading holistic therapies, due to its ability to assist in resolving many ailments, it is often used hand in hand with modern medicine. Added advantages are that it's non-invasive, easy to apply and an absolute pleasure to receive. The benefits of reflexology spread far and wide, whether received on a regular basis to ease symptoms or maintain good health, or even as a one-off treatment for relaxation. With no restrictions to its usage, it is a truly great healing tool. Not only can it initiate and accelerate healing, but it can also promote and maintain wellbeing and overall harmony.

How is this possible? Well, it's based on the principle that the whole physical body is mapped out, on a much smaller scale, over both of the feet. Everything, from the liver to the eyes to the elbows, has a specific reflex point or area on the foot linking it directly to the corresponding part or area of the body. Massaging these reflexes brings about an appropriate reaction in the body and this is when healing begins. The response can take the form of calming overactive nerves, stimulating underactive glands or easing tension, all of which helps the body to function as it should. Anything that gets in the way, such as negative thought patterns, long-standing hurts or troublesome memories, may be picked up by the feet and show up in the reflexes.

This is where reflexology steps in! Its main aim is to ease the mind, relax the body and reconnect with the true spirit, all achieved through the physical release of distress, along with letting go of emotional concerns and limiting belief systems. As this happens, muscles, organs and nerves can finally ease up and get rid of long-held tension. With the blood then flowing freely around the body, areas that were previously starved of essential life forces can once again be nourished.

Reflexology also boosts emotional and spiritual wellbeing, frees up innate gifts, enhances clarity of thought and brings balance, harmony and inner peace to the whole – mind, body, spirit. This is why reflexology is considered to be a holistic remedy. And that's not all! The effects of this massage are enhanced because the feet continually reflect fluctuations of innermost thoughts, uppermost beliefs, prevalent emotions and the state of the spirit. They do this by constantly changing their appearance, be it by altering the shape and position of their toes, or through differing conditions of their nails or through variability in the colour and temperature of their skin. Each unique nuance of the feet has a subtle meaning, along with an insightful message. Once aware of what feet are saying, it is possible to deal with the underlying emotional issue, by taking the preventative steps needed, before it upsets the body.

Massaging the feet encourages the release of resentment, anger, fear and other forms of irritability. It opens the heart to giving and receiving love. These are essential steps in the healing process, since toxic thoughts and noxious emotions are at the root of all physical symptoms and disease. Any improvements are immediately mirrored in the feet and reflected, through enhanced wellbeing, in the body. After all, wherever the mind goes, the feet follow. This is why reflexology is such a powerful aid. It recognizes that mind, body and spirit are all one and, for true healing to take place, all these aspects need to be embraced. Feet are so in tune with the mind, body and spirit that, by simply touching them, immediate improvements can and do take place. Reconnecting on all levels inspires individuals to put their best foot forward and keep moving towards greater health, happiness and fulfilment. All that is required is a willing heart, an open mind and the desire to make a positive difference for oneself and others.

10 Only got ten minutes?

What is reflexology?

Reflexology has been around since 2330 BCE and, for centuries, seemed to be common knowledge and a way of life throughout the world. Almost everybody intuitively knew how to massage feet and, in so doing, bring healing and health to mind and body, as well as revive the spirit. Feet have played an exceptionally important role in many religions. There are many ceremonies in which they are anointed, massaged and honoured, generally to signify the letting go of the old to make way for the new. Around 300 years ago, all this gradually fell away as the focus moved towards modern medicine. However it appears that, once again, there is increasing interest in this ancient form of healing, which has certainly stood the test of time.

How is the body portrayed on the feet?

Place the feet side by side and visualize the body in miniature, with the front of the body on the soles and the back of the body on the tops of both feet. The right side of the body is mirrored onto the right foot and the left side of the body onto the left foot. All the toes reflect the head and brain; the toe necks, the throat and neck; the balls of the feet, the chest; the insteps, the upper and lower digestive tract reflexes and the heels, the pelvic region. Every organ or gland has a specific reflex in the feet, which, when massaged, generates a reaction in the corresponding part of the body.

What reactions can be expected?

Reactions vary enormously. Once relieved of tension, the body can function more effectively and efficiently. Furthermore, getting to the root of the underlying issue frequently means that certain symptoms may get worse before they get better. This is the way in which the mind and body rid themselves of noxious memories and detrimental beliefs that repeatedly trip them up. Ultimately, massaging the feet has the remarkable ability to promote incredible life changes, which is why there is now far greater confidence in giving reflexology in any situation, from pregnancy and childbirth through to terminal illness.

Why is reflexology such a useful aid?

Reflexology alleviates a host of unpleasant symptoms, be they recurrent migraines, chronic digestive disorders, ongoing anxiety, latent diabetes or hormonal imbalances, to mention but a few. Many doctors recommend it, especially pre- and post-operatively, since it can effectively relax the mind and body, as well as accelerate recovery. Once the body is relieved of physical discomfort, there's greater peace of mind, which, in turn, restores the spirit. Reflexology is an excellent tonic for mind, body and soul. It should, ideally, be incorporated into everyday life and enjoyed at least once a week to ensure ongoing health.

How does it work?

Within everybody is life force energy that is essential for physical, emotional and spiritual wellbeing. It ensures inner harmony; that is until anxiety and concern get in the way. With the body becoming increasingly uptight and tense, the energy flow becomes increasingly inhibited and progressively stagnant, denying those cells that are further down the line their energy quota. This tends to really upset them. They draw attention to their dire circumstances through specific symptoms of uneasiness, which invariably cause the rest of the body to slow down, as it becomes increasingly drained of energy. Reflexology gets the energy to move and clears the way for it to keep flowing, unimpeded, throughout. Massaging the feet ensures that pungent energies are replaced with revitalized energies, making the individual feel so much better. Reflexology is one of the easiest and quickest ways to gain relief from physical discomfort and to restore energy throughout the mind and body.

What upsets the body in the first place?

All physical ailments and diseases are an outward sign of inner distress, concern or anxiety. Negative thoughts drain the body of its vibrancy; resentful memories create excessive anger; deep sadness evokes morose emotions; and limiting belief systems restrain and restrict the mind and body. The more the past is mulled over, the more the memory tends to grow out of proportion, until becoming a threat. The body eventually becomes sick and tired of having to deal with the same old tedious issue. Constant negativity, along with a hopeless outlook, darken the energies, making them increasingly dense, until they are bound to get in the way. The feet immediately pick up on this and change their characteristics to highlight areas of concern, in the hope that something is done to improve the situation.

So what can be done?

By getting to the root of the disturbance, Reflexology deals with it in the most appropriate way. With the reflexes being so intimately linked to the various parts of the body, immense relief can be attained through the loving and gentle massage of the feet.

Tuning into the more subtle, yet equally important, emotional and spiritual aspects of the body, encourages appropriate energetic adjustments to be made at the same time. This makes reflexology an extremely powerful healing tool. It accesses all levels of the mind, body and soul for true healing to take place.

What do the feet say?

Every aspect of the feet has an underlying message and meaning, which has become known as the 'language of the feet'. It provides incredibly accurate insight into the impact of detrimental subconscious and unconscious thoughts and emotions, the understanding of which helps to enhance the effectiveness of reflexology. As the soles are bared, the soul is bared and so reading and handling the feet always needs to be done with integrity, compassion, care and respect.

The importance of touch

There is no right or wrong way to touch the feet, especially when the impetus comes from the heart. The gentler the touch, the greater the effect; a concept based on the belief that 'less is more', which is the principle of the Universal approach to reflexology. Less pressure makes it easier to get a feel of 'what's afoot' and also eliminates any discomfort, especially on the more sensitive reflexes or areas. A variety of touches are used throughout a reflexology session, with the thumb being the most commonly used digit. However, massaging with the fingers has added another dimension, since each digit has its own unique energy, quality and contribution. Tapping and rotating a digit over a reflex eases mental and physical discomfort; 'milking' the reflex coaxes stagnant, stale emotions and feelings out of the way, while 'feather stroking' calms, reassures and supports the spirit.

A reflexology session

A reflexology session is generally around an hour. After a gentle
warm-up, both feet are simultaneously massaged to systematically
balance each body system, starting with the central nervous
system, since it calms the body and encourages overall relaxation.
The effects of reflexology last long after the session has ended,
as the healing energies continue to circulate throughout the body.

Reflexology round-up

Reflexology is a gift from the universe. It's a simple tool that
initiates healing and maintains health. Learning how to do it is
not only empowering, but also an opportunity to gain greater
understanding of mind, body and soul, as well as life in general.

Introduction

Here's the ideal opportunity to finally get people to put their feet
up and be pampered! With *Get Started in Reflexology* by your side,
you will be guided, step by step, through this incredibly safe, yet
extremely effective, form of natural healing. It really is an excellent
way in which to regain and maintain health.

There is nothing new about the concept of reflexology. It's been
around since humans first set foot on earth and so has most certainly
stood the test of time. Furthermore it is as effective now as it was
then. This book looks back at its origins, a fascinating journey
in itself, and shows how, since the beginning of time, reflexology
has served humanity as an outstanding and incredible means of
encouraging mind, body and soul to heal themselves. The information
shared here is regularly updated to provide intriguing insight into
the endless possibilities of this ancient therapy.

Meanwhile, the explicit instructions of how to massage both feet
guides you meaningfully, section by section, to reveal how, by
massaging the toes, a weight is taken off the mind, providing more
space in which to think; it shows how, by caressing the toe necks,
the very best is derived from the two-way exchange of life force
energies that enter and leave the body; it discloses how, by stroking
the balls of the feet, ruffled emotions are soothed and dispensed
with; it divulges how, by kneading the insteps, courage comes
to the fore in facing daily challenges leading to much healthier
relationships and, finally, it makes sure that, by rubbing the heels,
the most incredible progress can be made for ongoing success.

The great thing about reflexology is that there is no one way of
doing it. This means that the outlined procedures can be adjusted
and you can develop your own unique approach. Fortunately it is
very accommodating and it really *does not matter* if your attempts

are initially slow, cumbersome, inaccurate or confused. The body knows exactly what to do and compensates accordingly, so you can relax!

It is impossible to cause harm, even with inexperienced hands.

There are plenty of clear and concise illustrations to assist you in getting to know 'what's afoot'. It really is so fascinating to see how transient thoughts and inner emotions are constantly mirrored onto the feet, guiding you throughout the whole procedure. It's amazing to see how quickly recipients respond to having reflexology, no matter how well or ill they are initially, provided they wish to get better. Even if they don't, there is often a favourable shift to help them change their minds!

The soothing movements of the massage encourage vital mind-shifts, pacifying inner uneasiness, while the caressing movements have the most incredible knack of transforming fraught, uptight individuals into relaxed, easy-going and energized beings. Reflexology is truly remarkable! It encourages those who receive it to help themselves toward a more fulfilling, rewarding and better way of life. No matter how sceptical you may be initially, the effects of massaging feet are bound to impress you! They can be truly miraculous; so find out for yourself by putting it into action and make sure you find somebody to give you a treatment too!

You possess a very great power; the ability to heal yourself!

1

Reflexology at a glance

In this chapter you will learn:
* *how reflexology can help in restoring health*
* *about ongoing benefits*
* *its background and history.*

A brief explanation

Reflexology is a natural form of healing that is non-invasive, simple and safe to give, yet it is responsible for some of the most impressive reactions. It does this by alerting latent healing abilities within the body through the firm but gentle massage of feet, creating greater peace and harmony within – the most ideal environment for healing and health. As the reflexes on the feet are massaged, the corresponding parts of the body are either aroused or pacified, while, at the same time, tension is eased in the physical body, mental chatter is stilled and fraught emotions soothed. In so doing, the mind and body can reconnect to the essence of the true spirit. The welcome surge of vibrant energy that rushes through the body effectively flushes out energy impediments, rejuvenating the whole to such an extent that the body is likely to jerk with joy! This is followed, almost immediately, by a blissful state of inner peace that washes over the entire being, offering a much-needed respite from the chaos of everyday life.

Insight

Reflexology is a deeply healing holistic therapy that relieves
the body of disturbing thoughts and detrimental beliefs
so that the mind, body and soul can find homeostasis.
Massaging feet is so easy and an effective way of promoting
relaxation, the first step to staying healthy.

Reflexology provides the time and space to sort out the mind and
re-establish priorities.

HOW REFLEXOLOGY HELPS

The relaxation aspect of reflexology is important since it is only
when truly relaxed and at ease that mind, body and soul can
determine how best to regain and retain excellent health. At times
of not feeling so good, reflexology has much to offer since it
relieves discomfort from aches, pains or cramps. Its effectiveness
comes from getting to the very root of the issue, so that the
distressing memory associated with the symptom can be sorted
out and eliminated once and for all. The beneficial effects continue
from there. Fatigue, tiredness and exhaustion are counteracted;
nervousness, concern, worry or fear are soothed and undue distress
alleviated. In the process the whole body is cleared of impure
thoughts and toxic emotions, circulation improves, underactive or
sluggish areas are stimulated and hyperactive or over-productive
parts are calmed. This prevents any further drain of energy,
allowing equilibrium to be re-established.

Reflexology recharges the mind, body and soul, making them fit
for life!

Insight

Reflexology can bring instant relief to minor ailments, calm
deeply embedded emotions and bring about peace of mind,
all of which are essential for a balanced and holistic approach
to life.

Ongoing benefits

Once you are feeling better, reflexology is one of the best ways to stay in tip-top condition, but regular top-ups are required – ideally once a week – to keep it that way. A one-off session is great for getting back on track but it's staying there that makes all the difference. Reflexology is such a pleasant form of deep relaxation that caringly provides a welcome relief from daily strains, frustrations and irritations; it is so good for those receiving it! By rejuvenating and re-energizing all the cells, it increases vitality, boosts confidence and ensures a good night's sleep. It also re-establishes inner and outer trust, making it then possible to focus on what's important in life. With such an incredible sense of wellbeing, and feeling so complete, a more fulfilling and rewarding lifestyle is possible. Reflexology provides the courage and wisdom to cope with any perceived adversity and the opportunity to be authentic for ongoing transformation, growth and progress.

The aim is to keep getting better at being oneself!

Insight

Reflexology is instinctive. Think of a mother absent-mindedly massaging her baby's feet, as well as the relief of rubbing the feet at the end of a long hard day. Thankfully, no medical or academic qualifications are required to give a foot massage since reflexology is such an innate part of everyone.

Advantages of learning reflexology

There are many advantages to learning and giving reflexology, especially since anybody can do it, if they so wish. It can also be given anywhere, at any time, because all that's needed are your hands and the recipient's feet. Academic achievements are not a prerequisite and, although medical knowledge is useful, it is not essential. Furthermore, since only the feet are exposed, there is no embarrassment, self-consciousness or fear of feeling vulnerable. Painful body parts remain undisturbed, yet still benefit from the relief of having their related reflexes massaged. Also, with less skin surface on the feet than on the body, a more thorough and precise treatment is possible.

As you become more adept and familiar with reflexology you will soon realize that it has many far-reaching effects. It offers so much more than just an opportunity to massage feet. It takes mind, body and soul on an amazing journey that naturally comes with being blessed with a pair of feet. Reflexology is the beginning of a fascinating, enjoyable and rewarding experience; a process that is so inspirational that it provides even greater understanding of the intrigues of each individual's make-up and why everybody is so different. The massage itself generally takes around an hour, yet its effects last much longer, thanks to reflexology's all-encompassing and holistic approach.

Health and healing are only two feet away!

Background

When humans first set foot on earth their soles were naturally stimulated every time they took a step; the undulating, rocky surfaces kept them in good shape. That is until sandals and shoes came into being! Footwear immediately created barriers and, in so doing, diminished the foot's innate sensitivity. Today they still keep some people 'in the dark', making it difficult to adapt to what's happening 'under foot'. Reflexology replaces the impetus needed to get started and keep going. Long before shoes came into being, the importance of massaging feet was acknowledged, by virtually every tribe worldwide. At one time, this natural form of healing and health was alleged to be everybody's birthright, so much so that youngsters were taught how to do it from a very early age. This made certain that the knowledge was passed on from generation to generation.

> Feet symbolize mobility and security and are the foundation of the mind, body and soul.

Insight
Going barefoot and walking without the barrier of footwear naturally stimulates the reflexes of the feet, creating a powerful link between the energies of the Earth.

STEP BACK FOR A MOMENT

According to Greek legend, feet mirror the soul and any lameness was considered to be weakness of spirit. This is possibly why so many flocked to a well-known health resort in Delphi, until 200 CE, to receive reflexology, along with other spa massages, before retiring to a sleep temple. It was while asleep that certain memories came to the fore, bringing the foresight and wisdom to deal with everyday life.

Meanwhile, across the seas, in Ancient Egypt, the soles were believed to have kept the soul safe inside the body, so during mummification the bottoms of the feet were peeled away to set the spirit free. This also released the soul from its bondage and commitment to earth.

A great deal of attention was given to feet in the Far East. According to Japanese mythology, whenever Outo, a wise old soul, was questioned about his incredible healing abilities, all he would say was: 'See to the feet, my friend, and you have seen the body!'

Around this time, there was also an increasing awareness worldwide of witches, who claimed to absorb their mystical powers from the earth through their feet. This terrified the masses so much that, as soon as anybody was found guilty of practising witchcraft, their feet were immediately lifted from the ground. These are just a few examples of how feet have been viewed, revered and feared.

Use wisdom, knowledge and experiences to move on to the next stage of the journey through life.

Worshipping feet

The Bible has numerous references to the symbolic ritual of welcome and purification through the washing, anointing and massaging of feet. Reflexology is a furtherance of this sacred act. It too cleanses the body, with oils being frequently used to encourage the healing process. Today the feet of divine or eminent beings are still kissed and worshipped, as a sign of respect, a practice that was once common in most cultures worldwide. Even now, in certain rural areas of India, youngsters are expected to laud over their parent's feet as a way of showing their love and appreciation. Also in India, every year thousands of devotees, from all over the globe, travel to ashrams throughout the country for an opportunity to glimpse or touch the feet of devout, spiritual men, known as Babas. These devotees believe it to be their way of achieving eternal peace and personal enlightenment. Other ways in which they do this are by gathering dust from the Baba's footprints or by drinking water that has been poured over the Baba's feet.

All religions, arts and sciences are branches of the same tree.

The relief of it all

Since feet represent the roots and foundation of the mind and body, any form of restriction limits potential by tensing the body and feet. Being free of self-limiting constraints, however, relaxes the body and feet, which are then able to move on unimpeded; this is ancient knowledge. For centuries, various types of pain relief were tried and tested, but frequently the suffering continued or soon returned until they had a 'go' at reflexology. The twentieth president of the United States of America, President Garfield (1831–81), suffered excruciating pain after an assassination attempt. Despite an endless repertoire of treatments, his pain just wouldn't go away; that is until his feet were massaged and he got the immediate relief he so desperately craved. Reflexology shows absolutely no preferences when it comes to helping people 'get back on their feet'; it assists anybody and everybody, regardless of their position in life, skin colouring, religious conviction or social beliefs. All that's required is complete trust in the process.

No amount of pills or potions can heal the pain of non-acceptance.

10 QUESTIONS TO CONSIDER

1 *How does reflexology assist in re-establishing the health of the mind, body and soul?*

2 *Why is relaxation so important when it comes to healing?*

3 *What makes reflexology so effective?*

4 *When a gland or organ is hyperactive or hypoactive, what effects can reflexology have?*

5 *What are the ongoing benefits of reflexology?*

6 *Are there any prerequisites when it comes to learning reflexology?*

7 *How long does a reflexology session generally last?*

8 *What reduces the sensitivity of the feet? How can reflexology reinstate this?*

9 *What do feet symbolically represent in the body, as well as in society?*

10 *What happens to the feet when a person is uptight and tense?*

10 POINTS TO REMEMBER

1 *Reflexology is a holistic healing therapy with roots in many of the world's ancient cultures.*

2 *Reflexology is a gentle foot massage.*

3 *Massaging the feet relaxes the body and creates inner peace.*

4 *While relaxed, body and mind can better heal themselves.*

5 *Reflexology is perfect for reconnecting with the essence of the spirit within.*

6 *Massaging the feet deals with the emotional root of physical problems.*

7 *Reflexology clears the body of toxic thoughts, noxious emotions and dreadful memories.*

8 *The relief of physical symptoms is the first step to feeling better, which can be maintained by having regular treatments.*

9 *Anybody can learn to give reflexology and everybody can enjoy the benefits of a treatment.*

10 *The feet represent the mind and body's roots and their foundations, while forming a connection with the Earth.*

2

A complementary art of healing

In this chapter you will learn:
- *how reflexology complements medicine*
- *some helpful lifestyle changes*
- *about other complementary modalities.*

Modern medicine and reflexology

Orthodox medicine has only been around for approximately 300 years and so it is still comparatively young in relation to ancient complementary healing methods, such as reflexology. Being centuries old, they date back to when massaging the body and feet were accepted and expected ways of life. Today, thanks to medical research, it is so much easier to understand how the body and mind tick; it has made it possible for all forms of natural healing to keep pace with the constant changes in human needs. With medical knowledge making such incredible advances, reflexology can adapt and adjust its methods and approaches to meet each individual's needs. Many now recognize that the body doesn't just play up for the sake of it. Even Hippocrates, the acknowledged Father of Medicine, stated that the physical body reflects the tremendous impact of emotions, which, in turn, determine the disposition of the mind. He used to assess fluctuations in the body's humours to decide which course of action to take. This is also how reflexology works, and why, when used hand in hand with medical and surgical procedures, it hastens the healing process. Meanwhile the foot massage itself invariably brings much comfort and reassurance to the suffering individual.

Insight

Modern medicine is excellent for fixing broken bones and sorting out a wide range of physical disorders, whereas reflexology is ideal for accelerating healing, which it does by soothing emotions, relieving tension and accessing and dealing with the root causes of a condition.

Reflexology and modern medicine, when used well together, make a dynamic team.

Teaming up together

Reflexology can't possibly realign shattered or broken bones, but it can reduce swellings and inner tension, as well as ease pain and discomfort, creating the ideal environment for the bones to relax and settle back into their natural position. Modern medicine provides instant solutions to relieve physical pain and mental discomfort, making it an advantageous stepping-stone in providing temporary relief. This gives emotional and spiritual wounds time to heal. No amount of medication can ever mend a broken heart, yet massaging the feet can assist in finding the understanding and solution that lies within. Thanks to the more holistic approach and open-minded attitude of medical professionals worldwide, reflexology is now frequently prescribed, alongside some of the more conventional treatments. The results to date have been phenomenal. Combining reflexology and modern medicine has the advantage of integrating ancient wisdom with modern technology. By drawing from either one or both modalities, it is possible to take exactly what is needed to feel better about oneself and others.

Comparisons are futile because every body is meant to be unique!

Lifestyle changes

With more 'dis-ease' on this planet than ever before, there is no
doubt that the state of the body is a direct reflection of the content
or discontent of the mind. Health, after all, is the natural state of
the body, while 'dis-ease' is an outward display of inner conflict and
emotional turmoil, brought to the surface by current circumstances.
When a huge issue is made out of something relatively trivial then the
delicate balance between health and 'dis-ease' is likely to be tipped. It
only takes one unhealthy obsession, fed by the incredible temptations
of modern-day living, to throw mind and body completely off track
with the soul's purpose. These temptations, more than anything else,
take the focus away from what's important; they deprive the soul of
the ultimate joy of living a full and rewarding life. In the process,
self-esteem and self-worth become sadly impoverished through
constant self-criticism. As soon as health deteriorates, mind, body
and soul are left in a poor and unsatisfactory state, regardless of
wealth. Reflexology is the light at the end of the tunnel that can
help anybody climb out of this dark hole, to make worthwhile
lifestyle changes from which greater benefits and superb health
can be derived.

Overall health means complete harmony within the mind, body
and soul.

Other complementary steps

There are many marvellous natural healing modalities, therapies and remedies that can be used alongside or in conjunction with reflexology to enhance the healing process. For instance, the **Alexander Technique** realigns the posture in such a way that the whole body can re-energize itself, the effect of which can be magnified through reflexology.

Then there's the evocative smells of aromatherapy, which, when used to massage feet, add a sensual dimension. A popular **aromatherapy** combination that is often used to complete a reflexology session is a mixture of *juniper* to clear the mind, *bergamot* to calm the nerves and soothe the emotions, *neroli* to boost confidence and *ylang-ylang* to heighten the senses and create a much-needed awareness of innermost needs. Meanwhile, always keep a bottle of '*rescue remedy*' at hand to manage a panic attack or to break through persistent thought cycles that erode away at personal wellbeing.

Colour healing is an integral part of reflexology, either through visualization or through the use of gems and crystals. Both provide a means of energetically restoring balance, as well as retoning the body (see Appendix I). *Rose quartz* is commonly used in reflexology since it encourages self-acceptance. Gently place equal sized stones in the recipient's palms at the beginning of a session and leave them there throughout the massage. At the end of the session take them and lightly rest them against the recipient's solar plexus reflexes (p. 118) for as long as required.

Insight

Reflexology is even more effective when there's a continuous intake of healthy, energizing thoughts and beneficial emotions. This is because the state of mind can dictate the wellbeing of the physical body.

Herbs, well known for their remedial qualities, complement reflexology because of their incredible capacity to preserve health.

Also, **homeopathy** and **naturopathy** plant derivatives alleviate disease naturally and assist in prolonging the effects of reflexology when taken in between sessions.

Meanwhile integrating **music** into the reflexology session is ideal for reorganizing the body molecules in such a way that the whole inner structure has an opportunity to totally realign itself. This enhances overall harmony and establishes greater peace within (see Appendix II).

Reiki, the energetic aspect of reflexology, is used to shift and balance life force energies and replenish parts that lack vitality, hence the increasing use of the term 'rei-flexology'. Then there's **shiatsu, acupressure** and **acupuncture,** all of which clear the natural pathways for energy to access all bodily cells. A combination of reflexology with any of these can be really beneficial. However, whether used in conjunction with other therapies, or when used alone, reflexology always ensures that the very best results are obtained.

> Everybody and everything in life is essentially neutral. It's the intent that brings out the worst and best in people and things.

10 QUESTIONS TO CONSIDER

1 *How can orthodox medicine and reflexology complement one other?*

2 *What was Hippocrates' theory regarding the impact of the emotions on health?*

3 *Why does the body 'play up' from time to time?*

4 *What can't reflexology do?*

5 *How can reflexology contribute after surgery?*

6 *How can massaging the feet benefit mind, body and soul?*

7 *What exactly is disease and where does it come from?*

8 *Why is an individual's mindset so important?*

9 *What happens when other forms of complementary healing are incorporated into reflexology?*

10 *What role can reiki play in administering reflexology?*

10 THINGS TO REMEMBER

1 *Reflexology can be effectively used alongside orthodox medicine.*

2 *Hippocrates acknowledged that emotions have a noticeable impact on the physical body.*

3 *Reflexology is ideal for bringing comfort and reassurance during times of suffering.*

4 *Reflexology is very supportive of the body when orthodox medicine is the primary solution.*

5 *Reflexology can accelerate the healing process after surgery.*

6 *Physical 'dis-ease' is an outward display of inner conflict and emotional turmoil.*

7 *The state of the body is a direct reflection of the state of the mind.*

8 *Making beneficial lifestyle changes improves physical and emotional wellbeing.*

9 *Maintaining a positive mindset is paramount to good physical health.*

10 *Other holistic healing therapies that can complement reflexology include aromatherapy, reiki, colour healing, herbalism and homeopathy.*

3

....

Ease or 'dis-ease'?

In this chapter you will learn:
- *the importance of your approach to life*
- *what gets in the way of good health*
- *how to interpret symptoms.*

Your approach to life

You have a very special and unique approach to life, which, along with your attitude, determines whether you are emotionally in tune or in conflict with the environment. This, in turn, influences your state of mind and the consequential ease or 'dis-ease' of your body. When in good health you are calm, but alert, and up to any challenge. You are more likely to be on the lookout for worthwhile opportunities and show greater appreciation of the many gifts of life. In other words, you 'have a life' and are completely aware of the true art of living. Uneasiness, or 'dis-ease', on the other hand, is the end product of a long list of complaints and ongoing criticism, which highlight the internal discomfort of trying to live up to the ridiculous expectations of others. Instead of being true to the authentic self, both the mind and body become so far removed from the soul's purpose that intense frustration, complete bewilderment, incredible doubt, extreme unhappiness and emotional loneliness build up inside. All because of conforming to limited, often outdated and unreasonable belief systems that just get in the way of pursuing the many opportunities out there.

What it all boils down to is that terrifying memories, along with outrageous beliefs, continually plague the mind and body, causing a tremendous amount of 'dis-ease' and unhappiness throughout the world.

> Physical symptoms of distress are a sign of inner unhappiness and extreme dissatisfaction.

Reassessing your life

Whenever detrimental feelings build up inside, they invariably get in the way, causing excessive anxiety and unbearable tension. The more these noxious notions are contained, the more discernible they become, hampering progress every step of the way, no matter what. The physical tension is often too much for the body, especially when its scope of movement and ability to function become increasingly limited. Things can get so bad that there's a tendency to overreact to everything, even when knowing that the anger and impatience are completely misplaced.

> Symptoms of disease are signs that something is unacceptable.

Feeling hopeless and helpless just makes matters worse, and can even lead to the abuse of substances. It generally starts with food, since it's the appetite for life that's immediately affected, one way or another. This is why there is such a widespread misuse of food; it is the coping mechanism for many highly evolved souls, who feel like misfits, so they turn to food for comfort, or as a means of concealing their true spirits, or to protect themselves against being exploited. Next on the list is alcohol, frequently misused as a way of coping, either by drowning sorrows or creating misplaced bravado. Yet alcohol is a spirit that provides a direct link to the spirit and is a spirited way of celebrating life. Meanwhile tobacco forms the perfect smokescreen for injured feelings to loiter behind, when too hurtful to bring out into the open. Added to this is the squandering away of life on drugs, a way of desensitizing deep inner pain, as well as providing an often much-needed excuse for not facing or dealing with reality. Most people abuse something or other, to some extent, at some stage of their life. The good news is that no matter how bad things have become, health being the natural state of the body, it will do whatever it can to be healthy. Being pushed beyond the limit, when threatened in some way, or feeling completely out of place, provides a superb opportunity to reassess life and start again...reflexology is always more than happy to give a helping hand.

Insight

Step back to take an honest look at yourself and your life. Are you genuinely happy and fulfilled? Or do you hide behind pretence and addictions? Think of what makes you uneasy and then do something that makes you feel better about yourself and others. Your mind, body, soul and feet will certainly thank you for it!

Disturbing the status quo

Whatever disturbs the mind also upsets the body, causing varying degrees of discomfort. This determines the type of symptom experienced, which then invariably shows up on the feet. For instance, ulcers indicate that something that was done, or not done, is still gnawing away and eating at the insides, revealed by congested energy on the related reflex. Meanwhile, the pressure of constantly trying to avoid emotional conflict is enough to raise the blood pressure causing hypertension, which can lead to tension in the feet. Whenever sadness or remorse fill the body, the feet are likely to become heavy and be dragged through the motions of life. Also any deep hurts from the past that still burden the heart can make it uneasy and more susceptible to 'dis-ease'. Detrimental to personal wellbeing is an insatiable need for material possessions, usually a sign of never feeling 'good enough', which can show up in the 'emotional' parts of the body and feet. Then there's that one additional stroke of perceived misfortune that paralyses the body with fear, striking it dumb and bringing everything to an abrupt standstill; generally this is the end result of being overly controlling or from resenting others for constantly having the upper hand. An ongoing string of soul-destroying disappointments gets to the kidneys and their reflexes, particularly when feeling an absolute failure. The point is that illness does not just randomly pick any part of the body in which to create havoc; it is, in fact, the other way round. Chaos in the mind disturbs the related part or parts of the body and is reflected onto the relevant areas of the feet, especially when the issue becomes problematic. It's the body's way of showing that something has to be done to make things better. If there is still some confusion as to what's going on, then just put up the feet and turn to reflexology, because, regardless of the symptoms, it knows exactly how to sort things out both in the mind and the body.

Symptoms are a warning that the body is out of balance.

Insight

Reflexology can assist greatly in easing inner turmoil and offering extra support, especially during transitional times. Not only does it boost the body's energy levels, but also provides the strength and enthusiasm to move forward and make progress in life.

Reflexology steps in

Whenever there's a crisis, reflexology is delighted to step in. It knows how to deal with the uneasiness that comes from disturbing memories and assists in coming to terms with the traumas of the past, regardless of how devastating they may have been. For total relief from any form of discomfort, there has to be a complete shift of mindset and a favourable change of attitude. For instance, if constantly irritated by one thing or another and it keeps getting under the *skin*, then a rash or some other skin disorder is likely to appear. Similarly, when things consistently get up the *nose*, being continually bunged up is a possibility. Then if life in general constantly gets on the *nerves* then the chances of being exceptionally agitated, highly sensitive or very touchy are high, all of which can be aggravated further by lack of sleep or an unhealthy lifestyle. This can ultimately lead to a complete or partial dependency on drugs, food or cigarettes, all of which exacerbate the situation. The body shows symptoms of ill health until something is done to make things better for all concerned, which is an excellent time to have reflexology and enjoy its many benefits!

Whatever the mind believes, the body becomes.

Signs that all is not well

Sometimes sickness is the only thing to create an awareness that a massive change is needed to improve quality of life. There's always plenty of room for self-improvement! It's taking the first step towards a more healthy and worthwhile existence that starts the process of feeling better about oneself and others, as well as life in general. Consciously or unconsciously, there is a deep inherent desire inside everybody to be wholesome, well and balanced and the body does everything it can to make this happen. It has all the internal resources and inner strength required to get through anything and everything and it's extremely well-equipped to heal itself and stay healthy, if allowed to. Reflexology revives these innate capabilities, and once the body feels better, life improves dramatically. Being back on one's feet makes it so much easier to step ahead with greater confidence and to put the 'best foot forward' on the next leg of the journey of self-discovery.

Insight
All physical symptoms and diseases are signs that drastic changes are required for one's own good. Feet continually reflect what's going on at a much deeper level, so reflexology is the perfect tool for making much-needed changes.

> The body communicates through the ever-changing
> characteristics of the feet.

The remedy at hand

Reflexology is a great preventative tool. It can pick up and sort out disturbances in the mind, long before the body becomes upset. It does this by directing vital life forces through energy pathways, immediately dissipating energetic hindrances and flushing out mental and emotional congestion, all of which are physical manifestations of detrimental thought patterns. With less pressure on the mind, the body can relax and function so much better, as the surge of new-found energy infiltrates the whole being. Having said this though, when first giving or receiving reflexology, there may be a feeling of exhaustion and lethargy as old, stale energies that have been suppressed for some time, begin to surface. However, once the body's natural healing resources 'kick in', the feeling of wellbeing is so tremendous that no form of adversity, no matter how serious, gets in the way for too long.

> That which is retained is inhibiting; that which is released, heals.

10 QUESTIONS TO CONSIDER

1 *Why is your approach to life so important?*

2 *What can cause uneasiness from time to time?*

3 *How can resentment get in the way of wellbeing?*

4 *Why has the abuse of substances become so widespread?*

5 *What, in the mind, can determine the type of symptoms experienced?*

6 *How can blood pressure be detrimentally affected?*

7 *What can cause heaviness in the body and feet?*

8 *Why do some people crave material possessions?*

9 *How does the body signal that all is not well?*

10 *How can reflexology be used as a preventative tool?*

10 THINGS TO REMEMBER

1   Feeling at ease with yourself, your life and environment creates
    a relaxed and healthy body.

2   Being ill at ease, due to constant complaints, ongoing criticism
    or hanging on to unrealistic expectations can lead to 'dis-ease'.

3   Uneasiness comes from not being true to yourself or following
    your spiritual path.

4   Conforming to old and limiting belief systems can often get
    in the way of progress.

5   Food, alcohol, drugs or cigarettes are either used as coping
    mechanisms or as a means to reconnect with the spirit and
    celebrate life.

6   No matter how ill or unhappy, everybody has the potential
    to change their mindset and feel great.

7   Whatever upsets the mind upsets the body and is immediately
    reflected onto the feet.

8   For total relief of any physical discomfort, there has to be
    a complete shift to a positive mindset.

9   Being ill or sick can be a blessing since it is a much-needed
    catalyst for positive changes to take place.

10 Reflexology is a preventative tool that helps the body flush
    out any mental and emotional congestion, before they become
    a problem.

4

Who benefits from reflexology?

In this chapter you will learn:
- *about the benefits of massaging feet*
- *the reasons these benefits come about*
- *how everyone can benefit.*

Anybody and everybody can enjoy and derive enormous benefits from reflexology, since it enables each individual to find their own inner peace. The resultant harmony allows the mind and body to function efficiently and effectively which, in turn, raises the spirits. Reflexology is a non-invasive therapy that should be applied sensitively and gently to avoid unnecessary discomfort.

Be wary, though, of massaging the feet when there's a deep vein thrombosis because, as the muscles relax, the blood clot, usually in the legs, could become dislodged and travel to the lungs or heart, with the remote possibility of a stroke, pulmonary embolism or heart attack. Although there is no report of such an occurrence, it is still advisable to be cautious.

Reflexology is particularly beneficial when stuck in a rut, lacking direction, feeling alone or misunderstood or when constantly questioning, 'What on earth is the world coming to?' Reflexology can and does make a world of difference.

The effectiveness of reflexology spans every phase of life.

During pregnancy

Massaging feet during pregnancy (see also pp. 186–92) is enormously beneficial for both the mother-to-be and unborn baby, particularly when the approach is sensitive and gentle. Together they can enjoy this incredible time, which, after all, should be one of the most remarkable and best periods in a woman's life. With the mother-to-be's body relaxed, the constant flow of natural life force energies creates an inner peace and calm internal environment, with plenty of room for the unborn baby to grow and develop. This, in turn, reduces the risk of complications. Furthermore, with a livelier blood flow, both mother and baby are kept well nourished, boding well for a stronger bond of trust and pure love after the birth.

> Mothers-to-be and their unborn children thrive on reflexology.

Babies and children

Babies and children are energetically, and often painfully, aware of their parents' thoughts and feelings, so much so that their wellbeing is intrinsically linked. This is why, whenever a young child of up to 10 years old is sick, the parent, especially the mum, should be treated as well. Children mirror what's really going on at home, long before their parents are even aware that there could be a problem. Fortunately, youngsters generally love to have their feet massaged and usually respond particularly well, especially those who are ultra-sensitive. Reflexology is also really beneficial for hyperactive and attention-deficient children, who have such a hard time trying to conform. With greater inner calm, these youngsters can relate so much better to themselves and others. In this way, reflexology can help each child acknowledge the uniqueness of their own true spirit in such a way that they can grow into the individual they are meant to be.

Teenagers

Adolescents are well tuned into the universal energies, but are often reluctant to admit it for fear of ridicule and not fitting in. However, whether they like it or not, they do tend to respond incredibly well to having their feet massaged, especially when their minds, bodies and spirits need balancing at the onset of, and throughout, puberty. It also assists in the appropriate distribution of hormones, making them feel more comfortable about being themselves. Reflexology encourages greater trust and honesty in their relationships, assisting them in stepping into adulthood with greater assurance, improved tolerance and more poise.

Insight

Teenagers have the perfect opportunity to sort out their relentless and turbulent emotions through reflexology. Their feet can reveal the disruptive confusion that causes their minds to rebel against everything familiar. It's just a matter of getting them to agree to having their feet massaged!

Adults

Adulthood is a time for individuals to really get to know themselves and realize what makes them tick. The sooner they recognize that the only thing getting in their way is themselves, the sooner they get better at being themselves! Reflexology makes it okay to be 'out of the ordinary' and be extraordinary.

As self-induced pressures are relinquished, the wrinkles of concern and anxiety dissipate and, as hefty burdens and weighty issues are lifted from their minds, their bodies no longer need to sag in despair. Massaging the feet encourages adults to be more lenient with themselves and more tolerant of others. This minimizes the damaging effect of distress, fear and worry and restores their faith in life's processes. As adults become more relaxed, there's not such an intense need to be so much in control.

Reflexology puts people back into a much happier and healthier frame of mind and body.

Seniors

Reflexology is a wonderful gift to oneself when growing older. It comes with numerous advantages, such as keeping mind, body and soul agile and alert, while injecting the whole being with a renewed enthusiasm for life. As seniors become fitter, they rediscover their true meaning and purpose. Meanwhile, having their feet massaged is an excellent way of improving their concentration, so that they can focus on the more worthwhile aspects of life. At the same time there's a quicker turnover of tired worn-out cells, which can then be frequently replenished with new, vibrant and healthier cells.

Seniors who spring back into action can make the most of the rest of their lives.

Insight
Everybody needs to feel loved and cared for! Massaging the feet is as powerful as a reassuring hug and is particularly comforting when ill, confused, heartbroken or elderly. The gentle touch of reflexology makes everything seem so much better.

Distressed souls

Massaging feet when feeling unwell, upset or confused can provide instant relief. It's perfect for giving the boost required to start afresh. Reflexology meets the desperate need to be touched and cared for, while, at the same time, relieving innermost hurts, as well as any persistent aches and pains. Furthermore, it eliminates feelings of vulnerability or defenselessness and also dissipates any form of hopelessness. Destructive emotions and devastating thoughts become things of the past, enabling newer, healthier and rejuvenated energies to replace them. Having the feet massaged offers all the reassurance needed for the mind to clear, the body to realign itself and the soul to feel loved and worthwhile.

> Reflexology makes individuals feel so much better about being unique.

The family unit

Even if only one family member is receiving reflexology, everybody at home can benefit. This is because people who receive foot massage become so much more reasonable and a pleasure to live with. If the whole family is having reflexology or, better still, massaging each other's feet, the outcome is even more advantageous. The gap between generations is bridged, with greater respect and love being shown for one another. Everybody accepts each other for who and what they are. Each of them can then feel really happy about being an individual, belonging to such an understanding and supportive family unit.

> With peace of mind, a relaxed body and a contented soul, everything improves!

10 QUESTIONS TO CONSIDER

1 *How is it that anybody and everybody can gain so much from reflexology?*

2 *When giving reflexology, how can you avoid unnecessary discomfort for the recipient?*

3 *What makes it such a safe form of healing?*

4 *Are there any situations in which extra caution should be applied?*

5 *What are the benefits of having reflexology while pregnant?*

6 *Why should the parent, as well as the child, receive reflexology when a young child is sick?*

7 *In what ways does reflexology assist teenagers?*

8 *What gets in the way of good health in so many adults?*

9 *How can seniors benefit from having their feet massaged?*

10 *How can the whole family be helped, even when only one family member is receiving reflexology?*

10 THINGS TO REMEMBER

1   *Anybody and everybody can enjoy the benefits of reflexology.*

2   *Care should be taken if there's a deep vein thrombosis because the blood clot could be freed, through relaxation, and move from the leg to the lung or heart.*

3   *Reflexology is hugely beneficial during pregnancy since it keeps the mother calm and relaxed, creating a harmonious and nourishing environment in which the baby can grow and develop.*

4   *Babies and children are so energetically aware of their parents' thoughts and feelings that they physically mirror what is going on at home.*

5   *Reflexology can calm and balance overactive and highly sensitive children.*

6   *Teenagers who receive reflexology are better able to cope with hormonal changes, giving them greater self-assurance.*

7   *Reflexology encourages adults to let go of their anxiety, burdens, expectations and pressures, placing a new perspective on life.*

8   *For seniors, reflexology keeps their minds alert and their bodies agile.*

9   *Massaging the feet provides instant relief whenever upset, sad or feeling downtrodden.*

10 *Through reflexology, a family can be brought together with greater love, tolerance and understanding of one another.*

A closer look at reflexology

In this chapter you will learn:
- *the language of the feet*
- *how reflexology works*
- *about the condition of feet.*

Let your feet do the talking

Just as symptoms of 'dis-ease' reflect the state of the mind, so too do the characteristics of the feet. They accurately display the root cause of anything that is unsettling, long before it shows up as a problem in the body. This means that by observing the feet, potential problems can be seen and dealt with long before becoming too disruptive and causing havoc in the body. Yet, stress is still seen to be the main reason for illness; however it's not stress but *dis*tress that is so unsettling and upsets the body. Stress is, in fact, essential for personal wellbeing, keeping the body upright and the mind alert. *Dis*tress, however, makes things fall apart and prevents mind, body and soul from functioning as they should. The feet are quick to pick up on all this and immediately draw attention to the detrimental impact of unhappy thoughts and upsetting emotions so that they can be eradicated.

Insight

The soles of the feet reflect the state of the soul, highlighting areas of distress that could, in time, develop into a physical problem if left unresolved. So always take a look at the feet to gain some very useful, and often much needed, insight!

> The body speaks to its owner through the feet.

The condition of the soles

The condition of the soles reflects the state of the soul, so much so that whenever upset at soul level, the composure of the feet is immediately affected. For instance, when uneasy, the feet are more likely to become uptight and tense, while lack of energy causes a lack of substance, making it difficult for them to 'stand up' for themselves. Feeling off-colour drains them of their vibrancy, making them look rather insignificant and pale. Meanwhile, being trapped in a compromising or disadvantageous position or feeling temporarily disabled is usually a result of the mind being so contorted that it distorts the feet. If really severe, the feet may even come to a standstill. Feet, through their condition, reflect what's going on and draw attention to innermost feelings.

> Reflexology knows how to straighten things out in the mind, body and feet.

Literally 'at your feet'

There are many expressions with 'foot' or 'feet' in them, frequently used to symbolically describe an individual's standing and situation in life. When in a fortunate position, they are said to have 'landed on their feet', whereas being in a new situation, means first 'finding their feet'. 'Putting their best foot forward' places them in an advantageous position to make a good impression, but should they 'put their foot down' they could be taking a firm stance or are being obstinate! Then comes the embarrassment of 'opening their mouth' and 'putting their foot in it', or the pain of being 'trampled under foot' when their ideas are oppressed or treated with contempt. This is a good time to 'be on a good footing' with family, friends and acquaintances. Feet provide fascinating insights into each and every body, offering a basic understanding of unique requirements. Reflexology often brings out, first the worst, then the best, making it possible to really get ahead in life.

> **Insight**
> There are numerous foot sayings that reveal the role of feet in understanding overall wellbeing. For instance, constantly 'putting one's foot down' can cause rigidity, whilst 'standing on one's own two feet' makes for a stronger skeletal system. Feet assist in taking the first vital steps towards healing.

Feet reveal the story of one's life.

Get ahead through your feet

Feet provide a solid foundation, as well as the flexibility to move ahead and make progress. As the roots of the body, they offer all the security needed, along with the stability required to adjust to the unexpected ups and downs of life. From time to time, fear, uncertainty and anxiety invariably get in the way. As soon as self-doubt is experienced when 'unsure of one's footing', then the feet are likely to become less flexible, making the journey ahead more arduous and heavy-going – the chances of 'tripping over one's own feet' are much more likely. Once secure, content and happy about 'standing on one's own two feet', it's so much easier to get 'a foot in the door' and 'step ahead' with a 'spring in the step', adjusting to all the twists and turns of life. Life then becomes an exciting adventure of the mind taking the body and soul wherever they wish to go!

Everybody is headed for an unknown destination.

How reflexology works

The extraordinary and often miraculous ways in which reflexology rejuvenates, refreshes and restores cannot be fully explained, since, like any form of healing, it ultimately comes from the universe. To get an idea of what happens, think of the impact distress has on the mind, body and soul. Fear, anxiety and distrust can have such a devastating effect on the insides, physically, mentally, emotionally and spiritually, that the body instinctively defends itself. With further uneasiness and tension, the likelihood of adverse reactions increases with the muscles contracting and clamping mercilessly down on the internal organs and glands. The more the capacity to function is impaired, the more rigid the feet become, revealing the extent of this insecurity and uncertainty. The reduced mobility holds everything back, depriving the cells of their full quota of blood, starving them of their vital life force energies. The more drained and depleted the feet become, they more they weaken until they can barely hold themselves upright. With everything coming to a virtual standstill, it's so much more difficult to grow and develop. Instead potentially dangerous substances, such as toxic thoughts and noxious emotions, become trapped inside the body, causing further chaos. Feeling more and more overwhelmed and overly burdened can make the feet swell and possibly harden to cover up or conceal any vulnerability. This is a good time to help the body out through the feet.

Reflexology heals the mind, body and soul by subconsciously dealing with outstanding traumatic memories at a much deeper level to avoid any further emotional distress. The therapeutic massage dissipates tension, coaxing uptight muscles into relinquishing their intense grip so that potentially harmful substances are released. This immediately takes a weight off the mind, calms the emotions and lifts the spirits. With less pressure, the frazzled nerves are soothed and can function as they should. Meanwhile, as distraught emotions are calmed, there is a more peaceful internal environment, essential for deep healing to take place.

Sluggish, hypoactive glands or organs are stimulated and brought back to life through reflexology, while overexcited, hyperactive parts are calmed down. Either way the glands and organs can return to functioning far more efficiently and effectively. With increased elasticity throughout the whole body, it becomes increasingly flexible and mobile, which means that the blood can flow more freely and all the cells can be generously replenished and well nourished. The cells then have plenty of energy to rejuvenate themselves, making ongoing health possible.

Insight

Reflexology restores equilibrium by stimulating any sluggish glands and organs, whilst calming the more hyperactive ones. Once homeostasis is restored, harmony can resonate throughout the whole.

With the efficient functioning of the whole being, good health is ensured.

From the inside out

Reflexology soothes from the inside out and is an extremely impressive antidote to distress. Massaging the feet entices the recipient into drifting off into the most exquisite and deeply relaxing alpha state of consciousness – the tranquility enjoyed between wakefulness and sleep. By taking full advantage of this autonomy, the recipient can totally regroup and fully recuperate their energies. Their body is then able to completely rejuvenate itself through the ongoing formation of billions of new cells that keep everything in excellent working condition. When relaxed, the mind, body and soul are re-energized from two natural sources, the sun and the earth. The vibrant, light, positive male energies of the sun are soaked up by the hairs on the body, while the solid, dark, mysterious female energies of the earth are absorbed through the soles of the feet – reflexology increases this receptiveness.

As the vibrancy becomes utilized by the various organs and glands, the energy rebounds back to the surface, constantly changing the characteristics of the body and the feet, to create a greater awareness of what's going on inside.

Insight

Let go of trying to be in control of everybody and everything! It's a huge relief and surprisingly empowering. Freed from self-imposed burdens, worries and concerns, the mind and body can ease their tight grip on life and vital life force energies can flow freely throughout.

Knowledge is attained through positive and negative actions and reactions, with health being neutral.

A powerful relaxation technique

All perceived adversities, no matter how large or small, can either be a destructive or constructive force. It's a choice between being a victim of circumstances or being the victor, taking each and every opportunity and making the most of them. Reflexology provides the courage to overcome any perceived adversity, with the relief of letting go being so great, that it's much easier to get back on track with the soul's sole mission. Being an individual is the only way to get on and do something really worthwhile with innate talents; this brings about greater appreciation and acceptance for oneself and others. Reflexology encourages an enhanced quality of life. Being such a powerful relaxation technique, it is particularly advantageous in this frenetic age of relentless speed and endless deadlines. Maybe if 'dead lines' were called 'live lines' every body would feel less pressured and so much better!

For healing to occur it's important to go with, not against, the manifestation of illness and 'dis-ease'.

10 QUESTIONS TO CONSIDER

1   *How does recognizing and understanding the changing characteristics of the feet assist when giving reflexology?*

2   *Why is it so advantageous for the feet to reflect deeply disturbing issues long before they manifest in the body?*

3   *How do the soles reflect the condition of the soul?*

4   *What causes the feet to become so uptight and tense?*

5   *When do the feet become drained of their vibrancy?*

6   *Why does the shape of the feet become distorted?*

7   *How many foot expressions, such as 'getting a foot in the door,' come to your mind?*

8   *What can make the journey through life so arduous and heavy-going?*

9   *How is the alpha state of consciousness best explained?*

10 *Describe the personal choices available when it comes to getting better.*

10 THINGS TO REMEMBER

1 *Feet accurately display the root cause of unsettling memories, long before they manifest as problems in the body.*

2 *The condition of the soles reflects the state of the soul.*

3 *Feet provide a solid foundation from which to move forward in life.*

4 *Reflexology heals and balances the mind, body and soul at a subconscious level.*

5 *Underactive glands and organs are stimulated into action.*

6 *Overactive glands and organs are calmed and soothed.*

7 *Reflexology is a powerful relaxation technique that promotes a good blood flow throughout the body and ensures the optimum functioning of all its parts.*

8 *By inducing the alpha state of consciousness, the blissful state felt between wakefulness and sleep, reflexology helps the body to rejuvenate itself.*

9 *Massaging the feet releases the need of having to stay overly in control.*

10 *Reflexology encourages healing from the inside out.*

6

Body reflections

In this chapter you will learn:
- *how the body is depicted onto the feet*
- *what to look for*
- *the importance of both sides.*

Ongoing knowledge

Reflexology is based on knowledge that has been handed down, from generation to generation, for thousands of years. With the information having been relayed so often, over such a vast expanse of time, it's inevitable that the interpretation of the reflexes varies, according to each individual's understanding. This has resulted in a fair assortment of foot charts, which, although basically the same have in some instances, also been adjusted. The reflexes most affected by these discrepancies are the spine, ears, eyes, heart, breasts and knees.

Insight
There is such an assortment of foot charts, which can be highly confusing, especially when some of the reflexes are represented so differently. Yet everybody is unique, so each foot is unique! See the foot charts as guidelines and use your intuition – it knows exactly which reflex is where.

Also, many of the organs, glands and parts overlap in the body, which means that there can be a host of reflexes in a specific part of the foot. For instance, the nerves, blood and lymph vessels infiltrate the whole body, while the bones and muscles form the basic infrastructure, so all these reflexes abound throughout both feet. Furthermore, there is more than one way to access a reflex, either directly via the primary reflex, or indirectly through its secondary or indirect reflex, in line with the direct reflex, on the opposite side of the foot. For example, the primary reflexes for the breasts are on the balls of both feet, but can still be accessed via their secondary or indirect reflexes, on the tops of the feet (Figure 6.1).

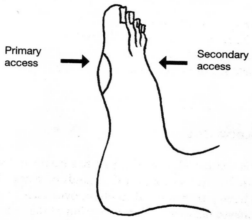

Primary access

Secondary access

Figure 6.1 The primary and secondary breast reflexes.

Picture the body on the feet

You can see how perfectly all the body parts are reflected onto the feet by visualizing the various organs and glands in miniature on somebody else's feet (see Figure 6.3, p. 44). The two feet together represent the whole body, with the front mirrored onto the soles and the back depicted on top. The right side of the body is reflected onto the right foot, while the left foot corresponds with the left side of the body. The accuracy of this is so great that, wherever a part of the body is missing or removed, there's a corresponding gap or hollow on the matching part of the foot.

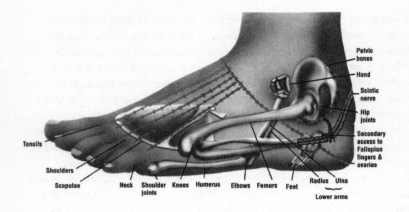

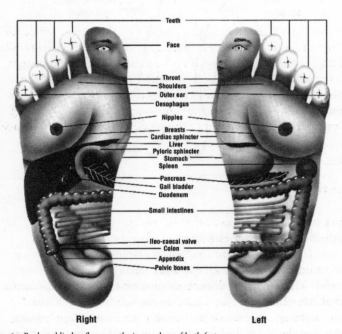

Figure 6.2 Back and limb reflexes on the inner edges of both feet.

Right   **Left**

Conversely any extra bones and organs always show up in their related areas, due to their energies, or lack thereof, rebounding back to the surface of the feet. Deep inner scar tissue is usually felt as a hardness, while bones that are crushed tend to have a shattered, splintered or gritty feel to their reflexes. It helps enormously to visualize the various parts of the body on the feet when doing reflexology.

To do this, visualize the body parts on a substantially smaller scale, as follows. The face is represented on the cushioned toe pads (see Figure 6.2, opposite), with each toe revealing a different aspect of the multi-dimensional mind. Notice how, more often than not, the big toes placed together resemble the shape of the head and face. Moving down the feet, the toe necks mirror the neck and throat, while the balls of the feet reflect the breasts and chest. See how their solidarity corresponds to the bony ribcage, while the domes along their bases together mimic the diaphragm. Meanwhile the abdominal cavity is portrayed in the fleshy parts of the insteps, whereas the denseness of the heels resembles the firmness of the bony pelvis. It's all there, on full view, so that you know where to place your fingers and thumbs when massaging the feet. By doing so, you can get a feel of what is really going on beneath the surface.

Out on the limbs

The upper surfaces of the feet are solid and firm, just like the back of the body, which they so accurately reflect. Marks and impressions from the past are frequently displayed here, drawing attention to unresolved issues that linger menacingly in the background. These include disturbing memories and unreasonable beliefs that have been unceremoniously shoved 'behind the back'; as well as anything unpleasant that took place 'back there'; along with persistent thoughts and feelings for anybody, who had their 'back turned on them'. A whole range of 'back' sayings highlight possible causes of *back problems*, of which there is an alarming epidemic worldwide. The more the past is dwelt upon, the more

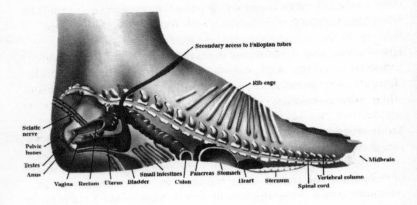

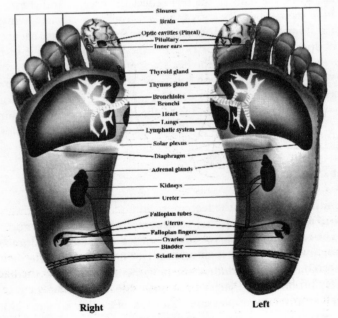

Figure 6.3 The reflection of bodily parts in miniature on the feet.

everything is held back, with reflexology being one of the ways to make the much-needed energetic shift to the present.

Just beneath the little toes are prominent bones that reflect the upper arm sockets, while halfway down the outer edges, of both feet, are bony protrusions, which correspond to the elbows. From these mounds take a 45-degree line to the outer ankle bones, where the fist-like mounds mirror the hands. The outlines of the outer ankle bones mimic the edges of the hip bones, from which the leg reflexes extend as shown in Figure 6.2 (p. 42).

The lower limbs are also reflected onto the soles of both feet, in the same seated position, with the knees bent up against the body (Figure 6.4).

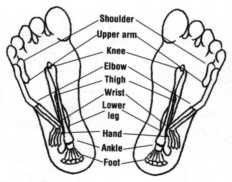

Figure 6.4 Limb reflexes on the soles of both feet.

Insight

The tops of the feet represent the back and the past. If puffy, then way too many memories or dormant emotions are being stored. With past energies dwelling so relentlessly in the back, any problem that hasn't been resolved can eventually cause back problems.

Either side

For the purpose of this book the term 'inner edges' refers to all the medial aspects of the feet and toes, on the same sides as the big toes, while the 'outer edges' are all the lateral surfaces, which are on the little toe sides of the feet.

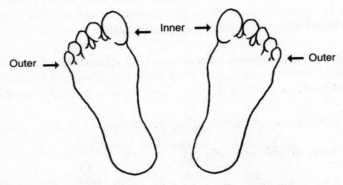

Figure 6.5 Inner and outer aspects of the feet.

Feet are perfect microcosms of the mind, body and soul.

10 QUESTIONS TO CONSIDER

1   *Why are there many different foot charts with varying reflex positions?*

2   *What's the difference between a primary and secondary reflex?*

3   *How is the body reflected onto the feet?*

4   *Which reflexes abound throughout both feet?*

5   *What do the upper surfaces of the feet represent?*

6   *What can be felt on the feet when a bone is crushed or broken?*

7   *Which parts of the feet reflect the front of the body?*

8   *Where are the limb reflexes?*

9   *What is the root cause of back problems?*

10 *Which are the inner surfaces and the outer edges of the feet?*

10 THINGS TO REMEMBER

1 *The primary access to a reflex is directly on the reflex, while its secondary access is directly opposite, on the other side of the foot.*

2 *The two feet placed side by side represent the whole body.*

3 *The right foot mirrors the right side of the body, while the left foot displays the left side.*

4 *The front of the body is depicted onto the soles of the feet, whereas the back of the body shows up on the tops of the feet.*

5 *The face and head are represented on the toe pads with each toe portraying a different aspect of the multi-dimensional mind.*

6 *The toe necks contain the neck and throat reflexes.*

7 *The balls of the feet represent the chest area.*

8 *The fleshy insteps portray the reflexes of the abdominal cavity and internal organs.*

9 *The heels display the pelvis reflexes.*

10 *The bony ridges, along the inside edges of the feet, carry the spinal reflexes, while the outer edges convey the limb reflexes.*

7

The power of your touch

In this chapter you will learn:
- *the way to touch*
- *how best to embrace feet*
- *the most effective ways to get results.*

The importance of touch

Your personal touch is the most important aspect of reflexology since your touch is unique. Nobody else can touch others quite like you do, so don't ever try to emulate anybody else – just be yourself! The recipient picks up on your feelings the moment you touch them; therefore always be conscious of where you are emotionally. Take in some deep breaths and centre yourself, before massaging the feet. Any form of caress evokes a reaction in the form of a sensation, be it conscious or subconscious. Aggressive, threatening actions cause the body to recoil or lash out in self-defence, whereas acts of kindness are reassuring and make life seem so much more manageable.

When giving reflexology, touch others with supreme sensitivity, the purest of intent and complete acceptance of who and what they are. The massage helps loosen and break down any fixation with time and, in so doing, releases inhibiting and intimidating beliefs, as well as haunting memories that have become a nuisance. The therapeutic movements of your touch can and do make a world of difference.

Making contact

Until recently the reflexology technique concentrated mainly
on the all-important physical and mechanical aspects of being
human. Now that there is more of a need to reconnect with the
emotions and spirit within, reflexology has expanded accordingly,
embracing all dimensions of the sensational and spirited being.
It has become one of the most all-encompassing therapies available.
As you touch the recipient's feet, you'll soon know how to tune
into their energies and innately know how to touch them, whether
it should be firm, medium or light. A general rule of thumb is that
those with a more physical approach to life generally prefer a more
definite, harder massage, although they often benefit far more from
the gentler touch; the more emotional and spiritually aware souls
tend to favour a softer, less physical massage, even though they
frequently need grounding with a slightly firmer touch. The desire
to be touched and nurtured increases during times of illness, distress
or insecurity, which is why the therapeutic touch is particularly
beneficial; it eases distress, pacifies emotions, reassures the soul,
induces confidence, creates trust and increases acceptance of oneself
and others.

Healing through your hands

When giving reflexology, use all your fingers, as well as both
thumbs, because each digit has its own unique energy. This alters
the vibration as well as the effect of your touch. It also introduces

a far greater range of healing possibilities, enhancing the overall effect of the massage. Your thumbs help in re-establishing trust and in creating a much-needed balance between the intellect and intuition. Your index fingers encourage the recipient to get in touch with their innermost feelings, so that they can be their authentic selves. Then your middle fingers activate their mind so that they know exactly what to do with all their amazing ideas, while creating greater awareness of their innate capabilities. Your ring fingers urge them to relate to new concepts that come their way so that they are courageous enough to communicate and share these and, in so doing, discover more about themselves. As for your powerful little fingers, don't be deceived by their size! They encourage the recipient to expand beyond tried and tested boundaries to become more of themselves, recognizing that they are unique and that it's great being so different from everybody else. All in all, your digits make an amazing team for bringing out the very best in others.

Insight

Always massage both feet thoroughly, regardless of what the issue is. A firm touch gets a response from the physical body, whereas a lighter touch calms the emotions and reassures the spirit.

For the best results

Whether reflexology is given to ease specific symptoms or to maintain health, for the best possible results, massage every single reflex thoroughly, with a combination of all four movements (pp. 194–7). Always pay additional attention to the brain (p. 63), spinal (p. 78), solar plexus (p. 118) and endocrine gland (p. 246) reflexes. Even though it may initially take an hour and a half to two hours to fully complete a treatment, with confidence and practice, this can soon be reduced to around an hour. Also spend extra time on congested, swollen areas or parts that lack energy and vibrancy, which are easy enough to feel. Resistance and hardness come with fear, anxiety or vulnerability, whereas a 'sucking' sensation is usually indicative of exhaustion or a need for some additional attention to help fulfil a deep longing. Meanwhile a dull, flat or unresponsive reflex is drained of energy and exhausted. On all these areas, lightly rest a digit and gently, but firmly, 'pump' the reflex until a gush of energy is felt. Alternatively, use the rotation technique (p. 194) to reawaken and stimulate the reflex. You will also be able to detect sluggish, hypoactive, or unresponsive areas that need reactivating, as well as those that are hyperactive or tense and need pacifying. Even if you can't feel anything, don't worry; the body knows exactly what to do, thanks to the impetus that you give it through touching the feet.

The best way of doing anything has never been found.

Always give credit where it's due

Whenever you trust your intuition to guide you, you will be amazed at the incredible results that occur before your very eyes! Within minutes there can be such great shifts in energy that, by the end of one session, the benefits are already obvious. Resist the temptation, however, to take credit for these phenomenal occurrences, since you are merely the conduit. Remember that the recipient, in deciding to get better, has used the universal energies, made available through reflexology, to help themselves to improved health. Not taking credit for the healing means that you won't lose confidence when, from time to time, the recipient chooses not to recover from life's events.

Insight
Those giving reflexology, or any other therapy, are simply channels and catalysts for healing. Ultimately it's up to the recipient to decide whether they subconsciously wish to get better or not. This means that reactions can vary considerably from being truly remarkable to barely discernible.

Sometimes this can happen when being ill and helpless serves the recipient more than being healthy; for the time being they prefer all the sympathy and attention that they can get! This does, however, tend to either slow down or block the healing process. Those who prefer to remain indefinitely incapacitated do so because of feeling inadequate or not being able to meet outrageous expectations. Resist the temptation to impose your will upon another, even though it would obviously be great to see them getting better. Sometimes they need to go through certain experiences, at a particular stage of their life, to get to where they are going, no matter how painful or long-winded these may seem. The best you can do is to keep them going through thick and thin by giving them regular sessions of reflexology.

Many see themselves as the victims of change and circumstances, instead of seeing an opportunity for growth and development.

10 QUESTIONS TO CONSIDER

1 *Why is touch so important?*

2 *Why should you approach reflexology in your own unique way?*

3 *How is it best to touch feet?*

4 *Why does it help to 'tune into' the recipient's energies?*

5 *How much pressure should be applied when massaging feet?*

6 *When does the need to be touched increase?*

7 *How does using all digits enhance the treatment?*

8 *Which reflexes, in particular, require special attention?*

9 *Describe the role of the thumbs and each pair of fingers during reflexology.*

10 *Why should you resist the temptation to take credit for the healing?*

10 THINGS TO REMEMBER

1   Your touch is unique so just be yourself and don't try to emulate anybody else.

2   Using all your fingers and both thumbs provides a far greater range of healing possibilities since every digit has its own unique energies.

3   The thumbs encourage trust and create the ideal balance between the intellect and intuition.

4   The index fingers assist in connecting with inner emotions and boosting self-esteem.

5   The middle fingers provide the courage to put personal ideas into action.

6   The ring fingers help in relating to new concepts and in communicating and sharing these with others.

7   The little fingers encourage the expansion of boundaries so that individuals can be proud of being unique.

8   Special attention should be given to the reflexes of the brain, spine, solar plexus and endocrine glands, since these all have a profound influence on the whole body.

9   Spend extra time on swollen and congested areas or areas lacking in vibrancy.

10 Always acknowledge that you are only the conduit for healing.

8

Foot characteristics

In this chapter you will learn:
- *about the healing qualities of colour*
- *what's left and what's right*
- *how one's angle on life can be improved.*

Take a closer look!

When doing reflexology, you have the ideal opportunity to have a really good look at the feet and observe any changes in their characteristics. The shifts can be really noticeable and generally happen surprisingly quickly. They will assist you in having a far better idea of where the recipient is coming from because of all that they have been through on their sometimes treacherous journey through life. Those who survive the most devastating circumstances and come out stronger for it often inspire others to do the same. They are also the best at extending a helping hand having been through so much themselves.

As far as a person falls is as high as they can rise.

Insight

The characteristics of the feet can constantly change throughout a reflexology treatment, as surfacing emotions cause them to shift their position, stature, colour, flexibility and temperature. All of these changes have a profound and important message to share.

In their natural state, feet are vibrant and pliant, making it so much easier for them to adapt and fit into the ever-changing circumstances of life. They are also quick to pick up on any change of thought or feelings. For instance, anger, resentment or extreme criticism rigidifies them, making them far more susceptible to injury and 'dis-ease'. It's when the past, along with a host of negative memories, gets in the way that endless frustrations are experienced. Whenever the going gets tough, the skin on the feet hardens and thickens in specific positions. These calluses or corns highlight areas of extreme susceptibility as well as protect or conceal true feelings or, alternatively, hide perceived inadequacies.

When giving in too easily under pressure or when lacking inner strength and substance to keep going, the feet are likely to become flaccid; whereas they tend to toughen up when going through a rough patch and needing to be extra resourceful. The skin on the feet looks shiny when there's constant friction or from continually being 'rubbed up the wrong way', whereas the skin flakes due to desperately trying to get rid of pesky irritabilities that keep 'getting under the skin' or from a 'flaky' approach to life. Whenever undergoing a complete change of mind or experiencing a total transition, the skin on the soles is likely to peel away as the old makes way for the new.

Be daring and think of what to change.

Colour

Feet are naturally flesh-coloured to comfortably blend in with the changing hues that colour the journey through life. Several different colours often appear on the surface at any one time but these can perpetually change as overriding moods and uppermost emotions fluctuate from one extreme to the other, sometimes in a matter of seconds. Some of the significant colours that appear on the feet are *white*, indicative of being absolutely drained, tired and exhausted, or as a sign of divine guidance and enlightenment; *black* or *blue*, from momentarily being in the dark and desperately needing an expressive outlet, or alternatively from being really hurt and emotionally battered; the depth of these colours indicates the severity of bruised feelings; tinges of *green* come from extreme envy or a profound need to just be; *yellow* indicates exceptional annoyance or a jaundiced view of life at the one extreme, while being overly conscientious at the other; then there's *orange*, which as a combination of red and yellow, often reveals mixed emotions about conveying something important, or else feeling really fed up and confused. *Red* is usually a sign of heated emotions, intense rage, extreme frustration, total embarrassment or surfacing passion; finally *brown* on the feet could be due to being 'browned off' or needing to feel more grounded and in touch with nature (or, of course, the feet may just be dirty!).

If only everybody would colour the world with their own brand of ingenuity!

Left and right

Energies absorbed from the sun and the earth are conveyed throughout the whole body providing a balanced view of life. While everybody has two eyes, two ears, two arms, two legs and two feet, it's the head, neck and body that bring everything together. The *back* and *right* side of the body are the connection with the past, while the *front* and *left* side of the body constantly reach out to the future; meanwhile the *central core* keeps mind, body and soul grounded in the present. By striding ahead, with one foot in front of the other, it's possible to gain a far greater understanding of life, with sensations coming from and being experienced on all sides. So when looking at feet, keep in mind that the right foot also reflects the impact made by men and anybody who is older; whereas the left foot is more affected by the presence of women or anybody younger.

This is balanced out by each cell having both male and female energies, with positive and negative input coming from dominant thoughts, uppermost feelings, past actions and immediate reactions. Favouring one side more than the other can have a detrimental influence on the relationship between the two feet.

Insight

The right foot reflects the right side of the body, along with past and masculine energies, whilst the left foot mirrors the left side of the body, as well as the present and feminine energies. The relationship between the two feet reveals how much impact past memories have on current circumstances.

Whatever happens on the one side invariably affects the other.

Taken from every angle

The angle of the feet signifies an individual's perceived position and bearing in life. This varies when walking, standing, sitting or lying. Every angle has much to say about the inclination to get on with life or the tendency to hold back. When walking, the feet should point directly ahead and be parallel, showing that the soles are on track with the soul's sole purpose. Being too open is a sign of being too accommodating due to a constant need to please others. Those who are pigeon-toed lack confidence or subconsciously wish to withdraw and go within, generally to do some intense soul-searching. Then the space between the two feet when standing reveals an openness to what's going on, as well as the scope of interest. The feet tend to 'stand to attention' when on their best behaviour or very focused or shut off for a while. While seated, the toes generally point in the direction of greatest interest, unless an act is being put on! When lying flat on the back, the feet should remain upright but supple. They turn or pull over to the right the moment the mind revisits the past and go to the left as soon as thoughts wander into the future. If the feet constantly change their position throughout a reflexology session, take note of this because it will provide insight into what's going on in the mind. Also be conscious of the recipient jerking, snoring or pulling a face; use this to gauge what could be going on at a subconscious level.

Insight

Observing the angle of the feet, whether on the move or static, reveals whether the soul is on track, as well as its openness to life. It also indicates the willingness to fulfil the soul's purpose, plus so much more!

The characteristics of the feet reveal the true story of one's life.

10 QUESTIONS TO CONSIDER

1 Describe the natural state of healthy feet.

2 What causes the skin on the feet to harden and become callused?

3 What makes feet flaccid?

4 Why do the colours on the feet vary so much?

5 List the meanings of the various colours that show up on the feet.

6 Which foot is more likely to reflect past issues?

7 What does the angle of the feet signify?

8 When walking, how should the feet be?

9 While standing, what does the gap between the feet imply?

10 How should the feet be positioned when the recipient is lying flat?

10 THINGS TO REMEMBER

1 *The colour of the feet changes as mood and emotions change.*

2 *White feet indicate feeling drained, tired, exhausted or enlightened.*

3 *Blue or black on the feet reveal being deeply hurt or in the dark about something.*

4 *A yellow hue indicates feeling fed up or having a jaundiced view of life.*

5 *Redness on the feet indicates heated emotions, frustration or embarrassment.*

6 *The right foot, along with the tops of the feet, reveals the impact of the past.*

7 *The left foot, as well as the soles, mirrors the present, showing its likely effect on the future.*

8 *The differing angles of feet portray the level of inclination to get on with life.*

9 *The space between the feet represents the degree of openness.*

10 *Feet change their position during reflexology, whenever there's a change of mind.*

9

....

State of mind

In this chapter you will learn:
* *about the toes*
* *about the workings of the mind*
* *what's at the back of the mind.*

Brain reflexes

Whatever is on the mind is immediately displayed on the feet,
especially on the toes since these contain the brain reflexes (Figure 9.1),
showing the content or discontent of the mind. Each toe reflects
a part of the head, with the right toes mirroring past ways of
thinking, while the left toes draw attention to what's currently
in the mind. Ultimately it's the nature of these innermost thoughts
that has a direct impact on the state of health and wellbeing,
revealed through the overall condition of the feet.

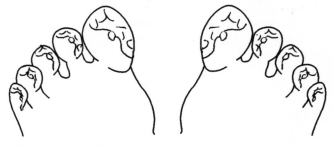

Figure 9.1 The brain reflexes on all toes.

Insight

The brain's activity and patterns of thought are picked up by the toes, influencing their shape, size and colour, as well as the state of their skin.

Looking at the toe pads

The toe pads mirror the face, exposing how well life is being 'faced', whether it's in a confrontational, bashful or shy manner. They reflect innermost thoughts and the confidence to face life head on with these ideas or a reluctance to do so. The *outer* edges, on the little toe side, represent the sides of the head, the characteristics of which are influenced by all that is heard within the family and society; the *inner* edges, on the big toe side, epitomize the centre of the head, where everything comes together to form core beliefs.

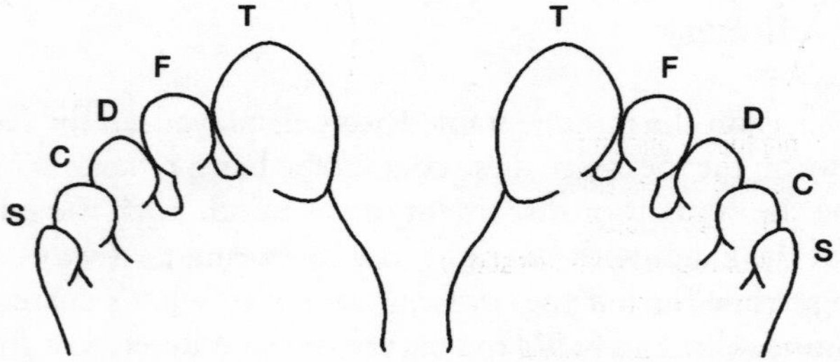

key T = thoughts
F = feelings
D = doing, actions and reactions
C = communications and relationships
S = basic security

Figure 9.2 Specific toe meanings.

Toe by toe

Each set of toes reflects a different aspect of the multi-dimensional mind and thought processes. The 'intellectual' *big* toes resonate to innermost beliefs, as well as intuitive and spiritual choices; the 'emotional' *second* toes are full of opinions about oneself and others; the 'enterprising' *third* toes have a wealth of bright ideas about what to do or not do; while the 'chatty' *fourth* toes reveal a host of views regarding personal relationships and the ability to communicate; leaving the *little* 'family' toes to disclose the amount of security felt within one's perceived status in life. Each toe can be visually divided into six horizontal sections, so take a closer look at each of these to gain a more detailed picture of one's mental and intellectual state.

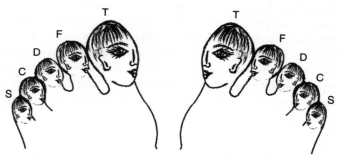

key   big toes = thinking
second toes = feeling
third toes = doing
fourth toes = communications
fifth toes = security

Figure 9.3 Facial reflexes and their meanings.

Insight

Massage the tips of each toe to help ease depression, irritability, vertigo, sinus congestion, headaches, insomnia and even baldness because the brain, hair and sinus reflexes are situated here. The calmer the mind, the calmer the body.

The brain, hair and sinuses

Along the tips of all toes are the brain, hair and sinuses reflexes, revealing the capacity to 'think off the top of the head'. The brain helps to reason, while the sinuses provide the space to think and the hair are the antennae that symbolize the power of the mind. When massaging feet, concentrate on these reflexes to soothe extreme sensitivity, ease intense irritability and increase the level of tolerance, especially when there's *sinus congestion, allergies* or fits of rage. Spend additional time on these reflexes for *baldness*, to reduce the need to mentally 'pull the hair out' and to ease the intellectual strain of constant doubt and ongoing uncertainty; for *depression*, so that light can be thrown on darker memories; for *dizziness* and *vertigo*, to stop relentless thoughts from spinning around inside the head; for *fainting*, to provide the inner strength to cope, even when everything else seems to be collapsing; for *headaches*, with the understanding that progress is still possible as things come to a head; for *insomnia*, to put the mind at rest so that the body and soul can follow suit; and finally for *nervousness*, to restore faith in one's own capabilities. The tips of the toes are energetically linked to the big toes, the thumbs, the fingertips, as well as the hands and feet. They are also connected to the nervous, endocrine and sensory systems, which is why massaging them is so effective in putting things into perspective

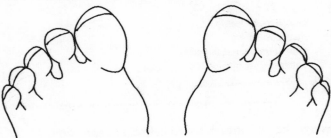

Figure 9.4 The brain, hair and sinus reflexes.

Forehead and midbrain

Stretched along the strips immediately beneath the tips of the toes (Figure 9.5), are the forehead and midbrain reflexes. These display the nature of deep thoughts, as well as the impressions gained whenever expressing one's own ideas. Favourable responses soothe and relax the brow, while 'frowning' on ideas causes the temple to wrinkle with concern; meanwhile intense disapproval furrows and divides the forehead. Spend extra time on these reflexes for *Bell's palsy*, for the courage to face the world as a unique individual, as well as for a *brain tumour* for toxic thoughts to be replaced with exciting new concepts. These reflexes are energetically linked to the toe necks, shoulders, wrists and ankles. They rely on the lymphatic system to keep the body open, through the constant drainage of impurities, as well as for the open expression of the mind and soul. Massaging these reflexes helps to clear the way for each individual to be unique.

Insight

Wrinkles anywhere on the body or feet indicate concern or worry. On the toe pads, they suggest anxious thoughts, while on the toe necks there is more likely to be a concern about speaking up and sharing personal notions.

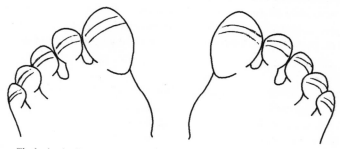

Figure 9.5 The forehead reflexes.

The back of the head and neck

The back of the head and neck are reflected onto the tops of all the toes, illustrating what's going on 'at the back of the mind'.

The toenails represent the skull and reveal, through their characteristics, the amount of care being taken to safeguard thoughts. Nails thicken when extra protection is required against criticism or mockery, or when desperately trying to cling to outdated thoughts and detrimental beliefs. *Vertical ridges* appear on the nails in sections that need to be particularly well safeguarded; while *horizontal ridges* arise at times of increased vulnerability. When a nail lifts or falls off, it's a subconscious attempt at exposing radical thoughts or of bringing innermost fears 'out into the open'. Those who tear at their toenails are metaphysically 'tearing their hair out' because of having no idea of what to do next; while those who resort to biting their toenails tend to be extremely anxious or uncertain about moving ahead.

Personal ideas and beliefs are also subconsciously protected from attack through the development of *corns*. If these appear opposite the toe pads, it's to stop ideas from being 'stamped out', while those that are on the toe necks arise from not wanting to 'get it in the neck'. Then there are those corns that occur on the outer edges of the little toes, as a result of continually 'turning a deaf ear', especially within the family or society. Reflexology gives the recipient the confidence to believe in themselves and their great ideas so that they no longer need to be shielded or covered up.

Insight

Toenails reflect the cranium, while their condition highlights how innermost beliefs and deep thoughts, especially those at the back of the mind, are being protected or concealed. Ridges reveal vulnerability, whereas the nail coming off suggests an intense need to expose radical notions or profound beliefs.

Belief systems

Social constraints and detrimental beliefs put a huge amount of pressure on the mind, limiting its capacity to think while

68

preventing full use of the brain. Whenever worried or concerned about what others think or don't think, or when fearful of the social consequences of doing or not doing something, there's a tendency to conform to unreasonable expectations that are no longer relevant. When this happens, the muscles instantly contract, clamp down on the cranium and put even more pressure on the brain, thereby depriving the brain cells of essential life forces. This, in turn, prevents them from functioning well. Further complications can arise when too terrified to speak up, causing loss of concentration, extreme irritability, great impatience, constant headaches, incessant migraines, increasing baldness, fits of frustration, distorted senses or exaggerated perceptions, all of which are signs of deep discontent. Reflexology frees the mind from inhibiting beliefs and encourages the full utilization of brain cells so that the spirit within can achieve all that it came to do.

Insight

Worrying about what others may think holds back some truly amazing ideas; it prevents them from making a much-needed world of difference. To make the toes 'stand up for themselves', straighten them frequently throughout the treatment. This increases confidence in sharing some extraordinary, but extremely valuable, notions. In time, toes can and do grow!

State of mind

The 'stature' of the toes reveals the state of mind, showing the degree of confidence in standing up and facing the world. In their natural state, toes hold themselves upright, yet remain pliant, firm and flexible. However, they immediately become rigid when set beliefs, an unbending attitude or an obdurate approach to life take over, invariably made worse by uncertainty and insecurity. When 'taking a stand', toes tend to stiffen with strong determination. They lean forwards, over the soles, to frantically try and get a point of view across, or when 'sticking the neck out', or when 'in another's face'. They 'bow' either from being subservient or going head first into life.

The toes tend to pull back, away from the soles, when withdrawing or holding back personal ideas, or as a way of avoiding confrontation, or to refer to something tucked at the back of the mind. The toes slant to the right to draw on ancient wisdom or when totally preoccupied with the past; whereas they lean to the left when drawn to the future or when a visionary. Reflexology encourages the recipient to face the world with their own unique and unusual concepts and reminds them that they came into this world to make a difference.

10 QUESTIONS TO CONSIDER

1 *Where are the brain reflexes?*

2 *What do these reflexes reveal?*

3 *What is mirrored onto the toe pads?*

4 *Which aspects of the mind do each pair of toes reflect?*

5 *When should the massage be focused onto the tips of the toes?*

6 *What do the forehead and midbrain reflexes display?*

7 *Which part of the head do the toenails represent?*

8 *What can cause a corn to develop?*

9 *Why might the mind be more pressured these days?*

10 *How do thoughts influence the stature of the toes?*

10 THINGS TO REMEMBER

1 *Each toe reflects a different aspect of the mind.*

2 *The toe pads mirror the face and how life is being faced.*

3 *Big toes reflect innermost beliefs, as well as intuitive and spiritual choices.*

4 *Second toes reflect thoughts and feelings about oneself and others.*

5 *Third toes contain ideas of what should or should not be done.*

6 *Fourth toes reflect thoughts regarding personal relationships and the ability to communicate.*

7 *Little toes reveal the amount of security within the family and society.*

8 *The tips of the toes reflect the brain, hair and sinuses, with the forehead and brain being reflected immediately underneath.*

9 *The back of the head and neck are reflected onto the tops of all toes; the toenails represent the skull and illustrate what's going on in the 'back of the mind'.*

10 *The stature of the toes, when flaccid or rigid, reveals altered states of mind.*

10

Toe characteristics

In this chapter you will learn:
- *how thoughts take shape*
- *about space in which to think*
- *the impact of thoughts.*

Shape

The shape of the toes draws attention to how ideas take shape, which, in turn, influences the shape of things to come. Toes change shape whenever thinking in a particular way or when there's a complete change of mind. For instance, *misshapen* toes disclose contortion of the mind as it frantically tries to fit into inappropriate ways of thinking; *boxed* toes reveal how so many amazing ideas have been contained, with a tight lid keeping them firmly in place for fear of the dreadful consequences should they ever come out; *pointed* toes indicate the tendency to 'go straight to the point', often with sharp, witty or, sometimes, hurtful comments; *squashed* toes are a sign that personal notions have been quelled, even before having a chance to take shape; *dented* toes suggest constant knocking of one's own ideas because of the belief that they are too inadequate or ridiculous. Reflexology helps the recipient to form a better opinion of themselves and others for a far better reality. Their life can then take shape the way they would like it to.

Size

The size of the toes shows how individuals size themselves and
others up, according to ingrained notions and prior experiences.
This then affects the capacity to think, with *larger* toes providing
additional space in which to play around with ideas, although
it could also lead to procrastination; *smaller* toes may indicate
a quick thinker who doesn't always take time to think things
through. Toes *shrink* when denied the opportunity to think for
oneself or when exceptionally fearful of what others may think.
Alternatively, toes expand and become *overly large* when bursting
with brilliant notions that have no perceivable outlet; it may also
imply that they are full of nonsense! To determine the ideal-sized
toes, look at them in proportion to the rest of the feet. Reflexology
encourages the recipient to think 'out of the box' and have a more
open and broad-minded approach to life.

Skin

When it comes to looking at the condition of the skin on the toes,
you are seeing the impact of conditioned belief systems and deeply
ingrained memories regarding 'kin', which determine the state of
mind. As the skin changes, it provides a fair idea of what is really
going in the deep confines of the mind.

Hard skin on the toes reveals difficulty in thinking in the same way as others; it *blisters* when there's a conflict of interests; it *shines* when resisting the opportunity to share brilliant ideas or when light needs to be thrown onto a particular situation; or it *weeps* when exceptionally upset. Massaging the skin smoothes things over while, at the same time, getting to the root of what's really going on at a deep subconscious level. In this way any disturbing memories that have been getting in the way can be dealt with and eliminated once and for all.

Insight

Yes, shoes are capable of causing blisters and extreme discomfort, but this can also be to create awareness of extreme emotional friction or uneasiness. By highlighting distressing issues, there's a remote chance that something is done to improve the situation, other than getting rid of the shoes! The position of the 'problem' unearths the underlying cause.

The colouring of the skin on the toes highlights emotions linked to innermost thoughts, showing whether loving, angry, hurtful, inconsiderate or caring notions fill the mind as explained in Chapter 9, p. 57. It's the essence of the thoughts that either enhances or drains the toes of their vibrancy. When there's more than one colour on the toes at any one time, take note of the reflexes that are being highlighted, since this will provide so much fascinating insight into what's going on beneath the surface.

10 QUESTIONS TO CONSIDER

1 *How much information can be derived from looking at the shape of the toes?*

2 *Why do toe pads change shape?*

3 *Describe your own toes and see if you can work out what is really going on in your mind.*

4 *What do you think the size of your toes indicates?*

5 *What can toe pads tell you about a person?*

6 *Describe the skin on your feet and then determine what it is telling you.*

7 *Is there anything you dislike about the skin on your feet? If so, why?*

8 *Is there any hard skin? If so, is it hard to be yourself, especially in the family and society?*

9 *What can be the cause of blisters?*

10 *How often do you massage your own feet?*

10 THINGS TO REMEMBER

1 *The shape of the toes reveals how ideas take shape.*

2 *Pointed toes reveal a tendency to get straight to the point.*

3 *Misshapen toes come from trying to force the mind to fit in with belief systems that aren't compatible.*

4 *The size of the toes reflects the capacity to think.*

5 *Large toes show a need for space to think and play around with ideas.*

6 *Small toes indicate a quick thinker or a reluctance to think for oneself.*

7 *The state of the skin on the toes reflects the impact of conditioned beliefs.*

8 *Hard skin reveals difficulty in thinking the same way as others and putting up barriers.*

9 *Blisters reflect a conflict of interests.*

10 *The differing colour of skin highlights emotions coming to the fore.*

The back and neck

In this chapter you will learn:
- *about the arches*
- *what gets on the nerves*
- *how to relax.*

The spine

The bony vertebrae of the spine (Figure 11.1) are reflected along the hard 'knobbly' ridges of bone that extend from the inner joints of the big toes to just beneath the inner ankle bones. It's from the spine that all the nerve fibres spread out, infiltrating the whole body and filling it with incredible sensitivity. This makes it possible to get in touch with innermost feelings and get a feel for others. At the head of the spine is the midbrain, reflected onto the edges of both big toes, just above the bony joints. The midbrain synchronizes all the body's movements, focusing particularly on the breath and circulation since it contains both the cardiac and respiratory centres. Concentrate on the backbone reflexes for all *back* and *spinal disorders*, such as a *slipped disc*, to put a piece of life back into place, as well as for *curvature* of the spine, to reduce the need to reach out for additional back-up when desperate. Massaging these reflexes renews sensitivity and reinforces ongoing support and backing. Reflexology ensures that the messages being conveyed, by the nerves, to and from the brain, to the rest of the body, are accurate, making it so much easier to relax knowing that the support is there.

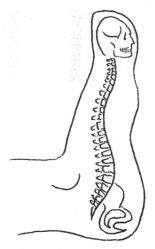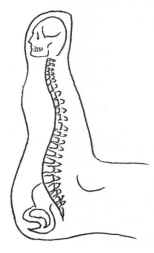

Figure 11.1 The spinal reflexes divided on both feet.

Insight

All back and spinal problems stem from past memories and beliefs that have been kept alive in the background. The past tends to hold everything back and prevent progress. So honour and release what went on previously by massaging the spinal reflexes, which will also boost belief in oneself and others.

The arches of the feet

The bony insteps that form the arches reveal whether 'in step' or 'out of step' with the general way of thinking and whether there's sufficient inner strength to go against the 'norm'. The arches are affected by everything put 'in the background' and anything 'going on behind the back'. This is also where the past resides, especially any grudges or 'unfinished business'. Most babies are born flat footed because of being so totally dependent on others to do everything for them, until they have the strength and confidence to 'stand on their own two feet'. Once the arches develop, the feet should remain stable and supportive for life, but the reality is that this doesn't always happen. They fall *flat* and collapse when immense emotional strain makes it impossible to 'stand up for oneself'; alternatively they become *overextended* to provide additional support during exceptionally challenging periods, or they 'bend over backwards' to please others.

> **Insight**
>
> Overly high arches reveal an extremely independent personality – one who rarely asks for help and tries to do everything themselves; or else it's somebody who stays in the background, preferring others to get on with it. Either way, ease the strain and help the arches relax through reflexology.

Reflexology is great at setting the record straight.

The nerves

The state of mind reflects the content or discontent of the soul, which goes on to affect the content or discontent of the body's composition. *Nervous disorders* are the body's way of saying that certain thoughts are 'getting on the nerves', so specific symptoms are used to reveal what in particular is making the nerves so uptight. Thoughts constantly run through the mind to the body and have a knack of jogging certain memories that, if filled with discontent, can initiate emotional havoc. A sense of feeling out of control, highly pressured or extremely anxious or just not being able to cope makes matters worse. This can immediately tip the balance one way or another, forcing the body to either overcompensate, in an attempt to get on top of the situation, or it just gives in, in complete desperation. Nervous issues arise from being highly irritable, on the one hand, or not reacting at all on the other; otherwise from being far too tolerant or utterly intolerant, due to being overly sensitive or totally insensitive, or simply from being tested to the limit. These extremes can have detrimental consequences on the functioning of mind and body (see Appendix IV).

When under strain, nervous impulses are more likely to become distorted or traumatized, with the smallest irritation sending them off at a tangent, causing an adverse reaction. This may come from a haunting memory that keeps interfering with the status quo until something is done to change the mind. In the meantime, symptoms of uneasiness or 'dis-ease' are likely to come to a head, since this is where the bad thoughts originally came from. Paying attention to what the symptoms are saying is the best way to determine the type of thought being triggered. For instance, *pain* is an outward sign of a grieving, anguished thought; an *ache* comes from an intense longing to be noticed as an individual; *tension* stems from extreme anxiety, frustration, fear or worry; *nervousness* comes from ongoing uncertainty that creates havoc in the mind; *infections*, *inflammations* or *high temperatures* flare up from festering dissatisfied thoughts; while *convulsions* erupt from fits of rage that distort the brain waves, throwing the mind way off course. Massaging the brain reflexes in the toes (p. 63) has an immediate effect on the nervous system since it instantaneously calms or excites, physically, mentally, emotionally and spiritually, depending on what's required. The resultant inner peace eases tension, relaxes muscles and ensures that the brain cells, as well as nerves, receive their full quota of essential life force energies so that everything can function well for the overall benefit of mind, body and soul.

Insight

Symptoms outwardly express unsettled emotions that invariably evoke mixed feelings. Whether there's an 'ache', an 'itch' or 'inflammation', the word itself reveals so much: 'aching for...', 'itching to...', or 'infuriated about...', so listen carefully to what the symptoms are saying.

The hands

Hands are handy for handling life, manipulating situations and moulding ongoing events, while fingers have a knack of dealing with the finer details. The reflexes for the hands are the soft mounds, in front of the outer ankle bones, on the tops of both feet (Figure 11.2). They feel like minuscule fists when palpated, while their appearance gives away a load of information on how well life is being handled. These reflexes tend to *swell* when overwhelmed at the enormity of all that needs to be dealt with; they *sink* when fearful or dubious about handling awkward situations. *Blood vessels* appear over the hand reflexes whenever feeling really unhappy about the way in which things are being controlled, or because of feeling so out of control. Massaging these reflexes helps to get to grips with all that's going on.

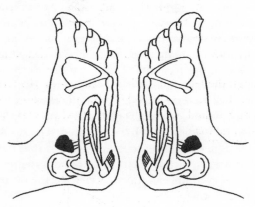

Figure 11.2 Hand reflexes.

The feet

Feet represent stability and security, as well as the ability to step ahead and make progress through life. They are reflected onto the lower portions of both heel pads (Figure 11.3), as well as onto the outer edges of the feet, just beneath the ankle bones (Figure 11.4). Their reflexes *bulge* when life is a drag or heavy-going; they *sink* when utterly exhausted from trying to get ahead. Massaging these reflexes is like giving a complete foot massage, without even moving your fingers from the minuscule reflexes, but it's not nearly as pleasant as a full reflexology treatment!

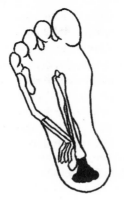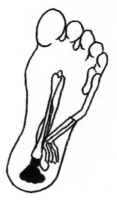

Figure 11.3 The foot reflexes on the heel pads.

Insight

Even though the feet and the hand reflexes on the feet are minuscule, they are important! The hand reflexes reveal how life is being handled, whilst the feet reflexes reveal the ability to step out and make progress.

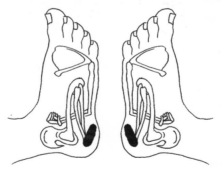

Figure 11.4 The foot reflexes on the outer edges.

Complete inner calm

Massaging the toes and arches has far-reaching effects because of their relationship with the nervous system, which means that every cell is influenced to some degree or other. Reflexology stimulates or soothes the nerves, immediately exciting or calming the corresponding parts of the body. More importantly, it encourages a change of mind and a far better attitude and approach to life. Keep in mind that each set of toes has a specific role, which contributes to overall wellbeing: the *big toes* balance the intellect and intuition for the confident sharing of innovative ideas; the *second toes* boost perceptions about oneself and others; the *third toes* inspire unique notions to be put into practice; the *fourth toes* help in generating new concepts for a fresh approach to life, whereas the *little toes* expand the mind, freeing it from inhibiting belief systems and social restraints, so that extraordinary ideas can make a world of difference.

Insight

Massaging the toes and arches calms the central nervous system, while soothing the nerves. This is the first step to easing discomfort or uneasiness that stem from disconcerting or disruptive thoughts, generated in the brain and relayed throughout the body. Reflexology provides the peace of mind required to move on!

Life is an adventure of the mind that makes the impossible possible.

10 QUESTIONS TO CONSIDER

1 *Do you suffer from back or neck issues? If so, where? Massage the corresponding reflexes on your feet and feel them ease.*

2 *Why is extra time spent on massaging the spinal reflexes?*

3 *When are the spinal reflexes stimulated and when are they soothed?*

4 *What do the arches of the feet represent?*

5 *What can be the cause of flat feet and overextended arches?*

6 *How does strain affect the nerves?*

7 *What impact do detrimental thoughts have on both the body and feet?*

8 *Where are the hand reflexes? What do they reflect?*

9 *Is it absolutely essential to find the foot reflexes?*

10 *What effect does massaging the toes and arches have on the rest of the body?*

10 THINGS TO REMEMBER

1   *The spine is reflected onto the bony ridges on the insides of both feet from the joints of the big toes (base of skull) to just beneath the inner ankles (pelvis).*

2   *Nerves radiate from the spine into the whole body, providing sensitivity on all levels.*

3   *Massaging the spinal reflexes renews sensitivity and encourages inner support.*

4   *The instep arches reflect whether one is in or out of step with general ways of thinking.*

5   *Flat arches suggest an inability to stand up for oneself, while overly high arches may indicate a reaching out for additional support.*

6   *Nervous disorders reveal that some thoughts are getting on the nerves. This creates irritability, strain, too much or too little sensitivity, while also affecting the level of tolerance.*

7   *Massaging the brain reflexes, on the toes, calms the nervous system and encourages inner peace emotionally, physically and spiritually.*

8   *The hand reflexes, on the soft mounds in front of the outer ankles, reflect how well life is being handled.*

9   *The foot reflexes, on the lower heels, as well as beneath the outer ankle bones, mirror stability and the ability to move forward in life.*

10 *Massaging the toes and arches soothes over active nerves or stimulates sluggish ones into action, balancing the central nervous system.*

12

The big toes and toe necks

In this chapter you will learn:
* *about the big toes*
* *about the influence of hormones*
* *different types of sensitivity.*

The 'thoughtful' big toes

The big toes contain the main reflexes for the head, brain, face and cranium, reflecting thoughts and ideas that are uppermost in the mind. They also reveal intellectual and intuitive awareness, along with spirituality and the connection to the Higher Self. The related reflexes include the neck, shoulders, hands and feet, which help to ensure that something worthwhile is done with personal thoughts and ideas. The big toes provide valuable insight into the nervous, endocrine, sensory and lymphatic systems, all of which are immediately affected by attitude and the approach to life. The element representing thoughts, because of its non-physical nature, is ether, while the colours are indigo, violet and blue, since these have the highest vibrations and are energetically linked with the divine source. Visualizing these colours, while massaging the big toes, provides space in which to think and connects the mind to its creative source, while giving it unlimited access to the universal library of ancient knowledge and wisdom. Reflexology encourages the big toes to realign themselves so that they point in the best direction to fulfil the recipient's soul's purpose on earth.

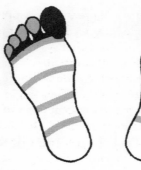

Figure 12.1 The big toes and their related parts.

Insight

The big toes are influenced by whatever is in the mind. Since they vibrate to the higher frequencies of blue, indigo and violet, any bruising reveals deep hurt around personal notions. All thoughts, however, especially the more extraordinary ones, ultimately come from the divine source.

In their natural state, the big toes and toe necks are superb springboards for thoughts and are in the ideal position to propel the mind and body forward to get ahead in life. The only thing that gets in the way is thinking that one's own ideas aren't good enough. This holds back the mind and body and adversely affects the big toes. Being far too terrified to stand up against 'authority', and being too scared to face the frightful consequences of being a non-conformist, compounds the problem. Anxiety, concern and worry keep tripping the mind and body up, while continually succumbing to unsuitable belief systems and being conditioned into prescribed ways of thinking makes the situation worse. The fear of not being in control results in self-righteousness or the need to be a control freak. Ironically, the compulsion to be in charge becomes more intense when so completely out of control – a no-win situation that drives everybody crazy! Nervous disorders evolve when thoughts have become so disorderly that they are no longer manageable, either because of being too controlling or too tightly controlled. Reflexology ensures that it's the recipient's unique ideas that propels them and gets them ahead.

Take time to understand what the big toes are saying. They *bend sideways* when side-stepping ideas, or trying to put them to one side, or from bending into unsuitable belief systems; this tends to crush the other toes, pushing them off course too. Sometimes the big toes *bow* in subservience, to please others, or to 'bow out' of facing the world with some extraordinary ideas. They might even *sink* into their socket when being pressured into succumbing to unfounded beliefs or from being 'under another's thumb'; they become *rigid* with very set beliefs and ideas that are generally incredibly out of date, resulting in a dogmatic or unforgiving approach to life. Massage the big toes well for all *nervous disorders*, especially those that literally stop the recipient in their tracks. Also for *gout*, to loosen rigid thoughts; *itchiness*, to release irritability; *multiple sclerosis*, to be less strict on oneself and others; as well as for *shingles*, to be less irate. Reflexology helps the recipient get their mind straight so that they can focus and stay in line with their unique and special way of thinking.

Insight

To locate the reflexes for the pituitary or master hormonal gland, place the two big toes side by side and determine where the centre of the head would be; this is where the pituitary gland reflexes are situated, on the joints of both inner surfaces. Massaging these reflexes creates harmony throughout.

Keeping the hormones in check

The best way to understand the endocrine system is to see it as the orchestra of the body, joyfully maintaining a harmonious inner environment and setting the tone for the whole body. The pituitary gland, in the centre of the head, is well positioned to be the conductor, directing all the other endocrine glands as to when and how to function, as well as when to slow down or speed up. Concentrate on these reflexes (Figure 12.2) for any endocrinal problems, as well as for *Alzheimer's disease*, to eliminate the constant need to escape life's harsh realities through leaving the mind; for *amnesia*, to erase the shocking memory that traumatizes the mind; and for *bruising*, to calm internal turmoil for greater acceptance of all that's going on. Massaging these reflexes assists the endocrine system in restoring inner control and in establishing greater peace for overall wellbeing.

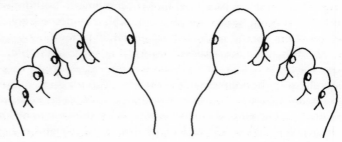

Figure 12.2 The pituitary gland reflexes.

Insight

Feeling out of sorts distorts the senses and reveals just how off track an individual feels. Sight, hearing, taste, touch and smell may either become overly sensitive or completely desensitized.

Sensory system

The sensory system makes known what's going on inside and outside the body, creating an awareness of the interaction between the two. Those in the healing profession tend to be highly sensitive, which can be advantageous when it comes to intuitively picking up on deeply embedded emotions and issues. Each of the senses affects specific parts of the body, connected to a particular aspect of life. This is easier to understand when you know which sensory organ resonates to which pair of toes and their related parts (Figure 12.3).

For instance, the *inner sense* is linked, via thoughts, to the big toes and toe necks; the *eyes* convey your feelings through the second toes which are reflected onto the balls of the feet; then *smell* and *sound* determine the type of reaction to whatever is done or not done, detected by the third toes and relayed to the upper halves of the insteps; *taste*, connected to the fourth toes and lower halves of the insteps, comes from the 'taste left in the mouth' after communicating with others, which has a certain impact on relationships; while *touch* highlights the amount of security within, sensed by the little toes and relayed to the heels. When uneasy, the senses tend to become highly susceptible, which distorts the perception of stimuli, either by magnifying them out of all proportion, causing various nasty reactions. This can result in numbness which means that the effect of the stimuli is diminished into total insignificance, so much so that there's no reaction at all.

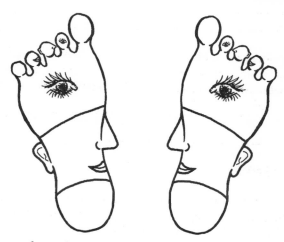

Figure 12.3 Sensory reflexes on the related parts.

10 QUESTIONS TO CONSIDER

1 Describe your big toes. Do you like them? Is there anything you would change about them? What insight can be gained from all this?

2 How does massaging the big toes contribute to the wellbeing of the whole body?

3 What is the natural state of the big toes and toe necks?

4 How might one's controlling tendencies be explained?

5 Why do the big toes require extra attention when being massaged?

6 What is the role of the endocrine system?

7 How does reflexology balance the endocrine system?

8 How do the senses contribute to overall health?

9 What are the various senses and to which toes are they linked?

10 Why is reflexology so effective when it comes to massaging the sensory reflexes?

10 THINGS TO REMEMBER

1 *The big 'thinking' toes represent the head, brain, face and cranium, reflecting innermost thoughts, ideas, intellect, intuition and the connection to the Higher Self.*

2 *The central nervous system, endocrine and lymphatic systems benefit from the big toes being massaged.*

3 *Ether, being the elemental quality of thoughts, influences the nature of the big toes.*

4 *The big toes resonate to the colours indigo, violet and blue because of their high spiritual vibrations.*

5 *The positioning of the big toes provides the thrust behind ideas.*

6 *Massaging the big toes helps to clear the mind.*

7 *Massaging the endocrine reflexes restores overall balance, control and inner peace.*

8 *The endocrine system relies on a healthy blood flow to transport the hormones to the target cells for appropriate utilization.*

9 *The sensory system creates an awareness of what's going on internally, as well as externally.*

10 *The big toes reflect the inner senses, while sight is linked to the second toes, smell and sound to the third toes, taste to the fourth toes and touch to the fifth toes.*

13

The expressive parts

In this chapter you will learn:
- *the importance of being open*
- *about responsibility*
- *about the need to be flexible.*

Down the throat

The voice given to ideas and the manner in which these are shared affects the neck and throat, which then shows up on the toe necks. The bony aspect of the neck, known as the cervical vertebrae, is reflected along the inner edges of both big toe necks, while the back of the neck is mirrored across the tops of all the toe necks. Beneath these, on the underneath surfaces, are the throat reflexes. They reveal the two-way exchange of life force energies that enter and leave the body, as well as the ability to convert non-physical thoughts into viable and acceptable components in the physical world. Whenever anything is done or not done with an idea, the repercussions bounce back, revealing the impact it's having elsewhere. The appearance of the toe necks discloses the openness and honesty with which things are taken in and given out, upon which healthy relationships can then be established. Massaging these reflexes creates a fair exchange of life force energies, which, in turn, ensures greater flexibility when turning the head to see every point of view.

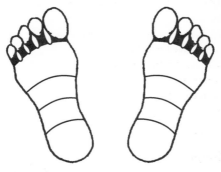

Figure 13.1 The neck and throat reflexes.

In the neck

When personal creativity is strangled or stifled by social restraints, restrictions and expectations, it can lead to anger, guilt or stubbornness. The fear of voicing unique concepts and 'speaking up for oneself' grasps the throat muscles by the scruff of the neck, effectively choking and throttling individuality. The dread of speaking up arises from an apprehension of being ridiculed; a fear of the possible consequences; a deep concern about outside opinion or the trepidation of upsetting others. Any insecurity or concern around self-expression tenses the neck muscles, reducing its agility, which can be a real pain in the neck. Whenever thoughts are threatened, the throat could go into spasm, while stabbing pains come from continually 'getting it in the neck'. Extreme anxiety and uncertainty about talking out of turn, but 'sticking one's neck out' anyway, can also cause severe tension in this area. Concentrate on, these reflexes for all neck and throat disorders, as well as for *cramps*, to ease the gripping fear of having 'one's style cramped'. Reflexology makes the recipient less twitchy by boosting their self-confidence and removing the fear of dire consequences.

> **Insight**
>
> When the toes curl, concealing the toe necks, keep straightening them out so that innermost thoughts, desires and emotions can be expressed. This is particularly helpful for a loss of voice, due to the fear of speaking up and saying what's really on the mind.

Neck and throat problems

When massaging the feet you may notice tiny *creases* and *wrinkles* around the toe necks; these are indicative of strain, concern or worry about speaking up or being spoken to in unsavoury ways. *Distinct lines* across the throat reflex occur when feeling throttled; while *lumps* and *bumps* are either collections of unexpressed emotion, if on the inner edges, or, when on the outer surfaces, a *post-nasal drip*, from not being able to cry openly. In extreme circumstances, the skin may weep from unshed tears. Concentrate on massaging the toe necks well for all throat and neck issues, to dissipate the fear of any perceived adversity; for *sore throats*, to ease the pain and strain of trying to disclose true feelings; for *laryngitis*, to calm inflamed, angry and frustrated words, left unspoken and festering in the gullet; for *tonsillitis*, for the free flow of individuality; for *glandular disorders*, to enhance the distribution of lively thoughts and ideas for the benefit of overall wellbeing; and for a *stiff neck*, to remove the blinkers and open the mind to seeing all points of view. Observe the skin's colouring (p. 57) around the toe necks for further clues as to what is really preventing the recipient from opening up and speaking their truth. There is a concentration of lymphatic vessel reflexes either side of each toe pad and toe neck (Figure 13.2), so milk these well to remove any congestion and open the way for free expression.

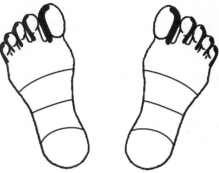

Figure 13.2 The facial lymphatic reflexes.

The thyroid gland

The butterfly-shaped thyroid gland (Figure 13.3) is reflected onto
the lower, inner creases of both big toe necks, mirroring a deep
desire to spread one's wings and fly, free of any constraints or
restrictions. These expressive reflexes become *distended* when
requiring more time and space to be authentic, while they *diminish*
from the utter despair of doing so much for others, leaving no
room for oneself. They tend to *harden* when it's hard to take
time out or when there's an ongoing resistance to personal needs
and suggestions. An extra layer of skin sometimes develops over
the thyroid gland reflexes to protect whatever space is available.
Massage these reflexes well for any thyroid problems, especially
goitres, to reduce the need to reach out to others for approval;
also for *hyperthyroidism*, to create more space for self-expression,
as well as for *hypothyroidism* to boost confidence and re-energize
the whole body.

Insight

The thyroid gland and its reflexes are shaped like a butterfly,
reflecting the desire to be free of unreasonable restraints
and social constrictions, which can ultimately interfere with

(Contd)

metabolism. Enlargement occurs when requiring more space to 'just be', whereas shrinking occurs when feeling exhausted or resentful from doing way too much for others, leaving little or no time for oneself.

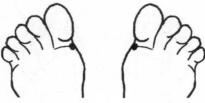

Figure 13.3 The thyroid gland reflexes.

The shoulders

Reflected onto the strips immediately beneath the toe necks, are the shoulders. These reveal an inborn ability to shoulder responsibilities, which are actually negligible, since the universe prefers to take the weight of the world on its own expansive shoulders. The shoulder reflexes (Figure 13.4) show the resourcefulness and willingness to carry on and overcome obstacles, even in the face of adversity. After all, being 'broad enough' to carry the whole body from place to place, they are strong enough to deal with anything! It's just when things become too overwhelming, from taking on far too much, that the shoulders start to complain. They really dislike all the many 'shoulds' and 'should nots' and may even *hunch* in defiance, refusing to take on any more. This is likely to cause these reflexes to *swell*, or alternatively give in and *sink* under the strain of needlessly lugging around such hefty issues. Massaging these reflexes encourages the recipient to let go of the overwhelming need to 'shoulder' so much, with the knowledge that the universe is always there to give a helping hand, no matter what is going on. The shoulders can then relax and continue with dynamism and fortitude.

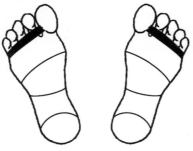

Figure 13.4 The shoulder reflexes.

The wrists

The wrist reflexes are immediately beneath the swellings of the hand
reflexes under the outer ankle bones (Figure 13.5), revealing the
amount of flexibility available in handling the many differing angles
of life, especially in dealing with others. Massage these tiny reflexes
well for any wrist problems, such as *carpel tunnel syndrome*, to ease
any distress arising from the way in which life is being handled.

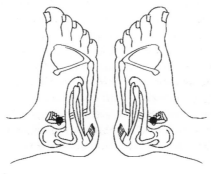

Figure 13.5 The wrist reflexes.

The ankles

The ankles assist in adapting to all those ups and downs that are invariably encountered on life's journey. To remain flexible and easy-going, they rely enormously on sincerity and truthfulness, especially within relationships. Massage these minute reflexes (Figure 13.6), on the outer edges of both feet, to enhance the ability to move freely, without any constraints.

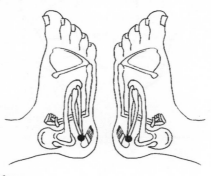

Figure 13.6 The ankle reflexes.

Insight

The suppleness of the wrists depends on the flexibility in handling the emotional aspects of life, while the agility of the ankles reveals the ease with which mind, body and soul are moving through life.

So what's in mind?

Reflexology reconnects the recipient with their reason for being. By preventing them from getting so caught up and frustrated by the mundane aspects of life, it creates greater awareness. In so doing, it encourages them to soar and reach unbelievable heights, particularly as their own astonishing concepts take off. This allows their neck, throat and shoulders to relax, so much so that they can enjoy some really meaningful exchanges and, in the process, create some much-needed balance and a deep inner calm.

Something that is being withheld makes the mind afraid and the body weak, until finding out that it is oneself.

10 QUESTIONS TO CONSIDER

1 Which reflexes can be found on the toe necks? What affects their condition?

2 Where are the cervical bone reflexes on the feet?

3 What can happen when true self-expression is being stifled?

4 What can cause the feet to cramp?

5 Which major body system is connected to the expressive areas?

6 Do you have any markings, lumps, swellings, etc. on your toe necks? What could these be due to?

7 What do the thyroid gland reflexes reflect? How does massaging these reflexes assist the body?

8 What effect does massaging hyperactive and hypoactive glands have?

9 Are there a lot of 'shoulds' or 'should nots' in your life? Where does this energy accumulate?

10 Where are the wrist and ankle reflexes? How does massaging these contribute to personal wellbeing?

10 THINGS TO REMEMBER

1 The toe necks reflect the neck and throat, along with the way in which thoughts are voiced, expressed and shared with others.

2 Massaging the toe necks encourages free expression, as well as flexibility in seeing different points of view.

3 Insecurity in expressing one's own thoughts tenses the neck muscles, causing rigidity and pains in the neck.

4 Tiny creases, distinct lines or bumps within the toe necks reveal limitations in speaking up.

5 Massaging the lymphatic reflexes on either side of each toe neck encourages the release of congested energies and frees up the ability to speak freely.

6 The thyroid gland is reflected onto the lower creases of the big toe necks, representing a desire to spread one's wings and fly free of restriction.

7 Massaging the thyroid reflex creates more space for self-expression and appeases the need for approval.

8 Shoulder reflexes, along the strips beneath the toe neck, express an inborn ability to carry personal responsibilities and any perceived burdens.

9 The state of the wrists reveals the amount of flexibility in handling life and in dealing with others.

10 The condition of the ankles shows the degree of adaptability when going through life's ups and downs.

14

The second toes and the balls
of the feet

In this chapter you will learn:
- *about ever-changing emotions*
- *how feelings affect the eyes*
- *about the capacity to breathe.*

The second 'feeling' toes

The second toes, known as the 'feeling toes', display thoughts of
self-awareness, personal views on life and opinions of other people.
They assist the mind in tapping into universal energies for enhanced
consciousness of a vast range of familiar, as well as unusual,
sensations. It's by experiencing these sensations that much-needed
insight can be gained into deeply ingrained emotions, stemming from
deep-set memories and beliefs. The spirit communicates with the
body and mind, through feelings, so that there's greater awareness of
the essence within. Feelings are also the link, through the breath, with
all that's going on in the immediate vicinity and literally 'hang in the
air' contributing to the emotional environment. With every breath,
a fair amount of air is taken in, packed with the emotions of
everybody nearby; a thought that can be either really reassuring
or extremely disturbing! The lungs then process and assimilate
these mixed feelings, and add emotions 'kept close to the chest',
before exhaling. This new blend of feelings fills the atmospheric air,
affecting anybody nearby, to some extent or other, which is why

occasionally it feels like 'the atmosphere could have been cut with a knife'.

Insight

The characteristics of the second toes are affected by feelings of self-worth and self-esteem, which is influenced by the parents. The impact this has is mirrored through the condition of the respiratory system, breasts and circulatory systems, all of which are reflected onto the balls of the feet.

It's through the breath that the second toes are directly linked to the respiratory system and indirectly connected to the heart and circulation. These toes are also energetically associated with the eyes, index fingers, bottom halves of the lower arms and shins, as well as the breasts and chest; the latter are displayed on the balls of the feet. Problems with the second toes highlight issues regarding self-esteem, generally affected by the father's circumstances during the more formative years and the ongoing relationship with him. A poor self-esteem can stem from never having gained his full approval. Gently squeezing the second toes releases these distressing thoughts, with the knowledge that memories can be changed when seen from a different point of view; this can then create a far more harmonious and accepting emotional environment.

Reflexology encourages individuals to like themselves and others better.

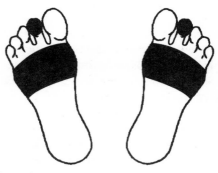

Figure 14.1 The second toes and related parts.

Emotions

The word 'emotion' comes from 'energy in motion'; the 'energy' being 'thoughts' and the 'motion' their movement as they are run through the body. The motion of the energy arouses deep memories and unlocks suppressed feelings, which, when liberated, bring out repressed, once-inhibited, aspects of the spirit. It is these feelings that provide the impetus to act and react, according to what's going on, or not going on, emotionally. Emotions are exceptionally powerful; when used constructively, they inspire and motivate the spirit, evoking compassion, empathy and pure love. They are a vital part of being human and contribute greatly towards being a unique individual, as well as to personal wellbeing.

The essence of emotions 'kept close to the chest' is mirrored onto the balls of the feet. The colours linked to them are green and pink, while the element that gives feelings a free range is air. Emotions left 'hanging in the air' affect both the internal and external environments of the mind, body and soul. So it is that any air in the body represents emotions, be it through *belching* or *farting*, both of which are natural ways of releasing stale emotions. *Air embolisms* come from a gradual build-up of hurt emotions that eventually get in the way and can bring things to a standstill. Reflexology allows the recipient to relish the emotion while it is still relevant, but moves it on as soon as it is no longer valid.

Insight

Thoughts are an energy that constantly 'run' through the body. These barely discernible movements cause minuscule vibrations that stir the cells, arousing dormant feelings and suppressed memories. This often causes confusion as to where certain 'emotions' (energy in motion) come from.

Feeling good is the soul's way of shouting 'This is who I am!'

The eyes

The eye reflexes (Figure 14.2), together with the pineal gland reflexes, can be found on the central mounds of all toe pads. They are ideally situated for innermost feelings to become evident when looking deep into the eyes. After all, the eyes are the windows to the soul and, as such, reflect the true essence of the spirit. They assist in focusing on specific aspects of life, adapting a multitude of light waves into meaningful shapes, so that life is so much clearer. The eyes are energetically allied to the second toes and all its associates, making them extremely sensitive to any shift in emotion. Every part of the body is influenced by what is seen or not seen, depending on thoughts and feelings that are currently emerging. Spend time massaging these reflexes for any eye disorder, including *blindness*, preventing the need to 'turn a blind eye'; *cataracts*, for the bigger picture to be seen more clearly; *coma*, for the truth to come to light; *conjunctivitis*, to make everything in sight more acceptable; *dry eyes*, to allow the true meaning of life to flow before the eyes; *glaucoma*, to replace set views with greater foresight, and for *tunnel vision*, to broaden the outlook. Rub the eye reflexes to open the eyes to the many exciting possibilities that are in sight.

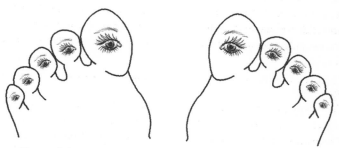

Figure 14.2 The eye reflexes.

Insight

The eyes only see what the mind is prepared to comprehend, but whatever they see evokes a thought, based on a memory

(Contd)

that then stirs an emotion. This affects the breath, with either a gasp of fear or a deep sigh of gratitude. The eye reflexes, in the centres of each toe pad are, therefore, linked to the balls of the feet, which contain the lung and breast reflexes.

The eyes reveal the antiquity of the soul.

The insightful inner tutor

Although the *pineal gland* (Figure 14.3) shares the same reflexes as the pituitary gland, it responds particularly well to the eye reflexes being massaged since these are their secondary access. The eyes influence the quantity and quality of melatonin produced by the pineal gland, according to the amount of light entering the body, which is why their state and condition is of utmost importance for the pineal gland's wellbeing. Through the eyes, the pineal gland controls all natural cycles, such as mood cycles, sleep cycles and menstrual cycles, all of which are affected by the emotions, as well as one's perceptions of life, making this gland either function incredibly well or go way out of control. Focus on these reflexes for *addictive* personalities, experiencing extreme difficulty in fitting in and conforming; also for *cancer*, to minimize any growing resentment. Massaging the pineal gland reflexes eases congested emotions and makes way for extraordinary insight and greater compassion. It helps the recipient to become increasingly intuitive and insightful with each natural cycle.

Insight

The pineal gland, or third eye, provides a balanced, intuitive and sensitive perception of life. Overwhelming distrust, fear and anxiety tend to cause extreme uncertainty, darkness and depression. Massaging these reflexes makes it easier to tune into the cycles of life for greater insight into family and relationships, as well as what is going on, especially regarding feelings and thoughts.

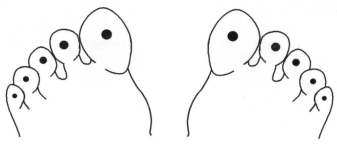

Figure 14.3 The pineal gland reflexes.

The balls of the feet

The balls of the feet contain the reflexes for the chest, breast, ribcage, lungs, thymus gland, upper arm, airway and oesophagus, all of which reflect the impact that feelings have on personal wellbeing. This then determines the type of reaction and response to constant changes and fluctuations within the emotional environment. The balls of the feet are naturally flexible, while their colour mirrors the ability to comfortably adapt and blend into whatever's going on emotionally in the immediate vicinity. They put a spring in the step, when happy, keeping mind and body buoyant or they can make life heavy-going when feeling down. Massage the balls of the feet for a quick boost to the morale; also give them extra attention for any emotional congestion, so that the muscles can relax and life force energies can flow more freely to shift any stagnant feelings; for *anorexia*, to bolster the flagging spirit; for *belching*, to calm inner panic; for *cancer*, to help resolve dormant sadness; for *cysts*, to remove the need for pity due to perceived ongoing misfortune; for *gangrene*, to restore the desire to be alive; for *pain*, to let go of feelings of inadequacy and hurt stemming from unfair criticism; for *snoring*, to finally be rid of deep-seated emotions and, finally, for *wounds*, to heal injured emotions. Reflexology restores belief in oneself and others, injecting the whole being with such enthusiasm that it's impossible not to feel happy and good about oneself again.

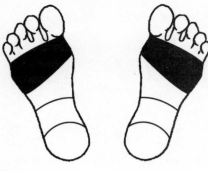

Figure 14.4 The balls of the feet.

Feelings vibrate throughout the whole being bringing it to life!

Insight

The balls of the feet reflect the chest area, lungs and heart, as well as innermost emotions and deep feelings. Hard skin is likely to develop when a protection or barrier is required to prevent getting hurt or from being taken advantage of.

Fluctuating emotions

The balls of the feet frequently change colour to portray fluctuating emotions. As memories flood to the surface, there's a mottled picture of past incidents caused by incredible uneasiness. As you massage the feet, notice these changes in colour as detailed in Chapter 8, and also look at the facial expressions as shifts occur. The balls of the feet carry the marks of heartfelt issues that have had the greatest impact, such as a *line* down the centre that appears when emotionally 'drawing the line' to survive, or when torn apart by divided loyalties. *Hard skin* and *calluses* are common here to either conceal deep feelings or provide protection, especially when feeling particularly helpless or extremely vulnerable. Reflexology helps the recipient feel so much better about everything.

> Nobody can choose how they feel, but they can choose what to do about it.

The lungs

The lung reflexes (Figure 14.5) occupy the bulk of the balls of the feet, both top and bottom. They represent the ability to expand and become more of oneself using bigger and deeper breaths to boost confidence. In this way anything can be confronted, regardless of the emotions being evoked. The breath is frequently used to suppress or express disturbing and unpleasant emotions, while the lungs reveal the overall capacity to do this. Constant interference with this process, because of not being able to cope, may cause the balls of the feet to swell and seem *engorged*. At the other extreme is giving too much of oneself to compensate for perceived inadequacies, causing the balls of the feet *flatten*; a true sign of feeling winded and deflated. These reflexes often *wrinkle* when constantly concerned about upsetting other people, even though emotionally distraught oneself. Excite the lung reflexes to give the recipient the courage to be themselves.

Insight

Conflict between the mind and heart immediately affects the breath, making it difficult to breathe. Massaging the lung reflexes, on the balls of the feet, eases this and enhances the capacity to live life to the full.

Breathing and respiratory problems

Breathing problems and respiratory disorders occur when interest in life has diminished or when feeling totally inadequate, unappreciated, when disillusioned or emotionally deflated, usually around personal relationships with the father or

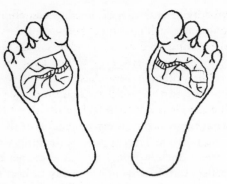

Figure 14.5 The lung reflexes.

dominant male figure. The temptation to keep heartfelt feelings 'close to the chest' or hide true sentiments behind a smokescreen, can eventually make it really difficult to breathe. Soothe the respiratory reflexes for all respiratory disorders, including *asphyxiating attacks*, to ease inner panic; for *asthma*, to alleviate anxiety, making it easier to breathe; for *chest congestion*, to shift emotional obstacles; for *emphysema*, to boost feelings of self-worth; for *hyperventilation*, to create inner calm; and for *pneumonia*, to encourage emotional hurts to heal. Reflexology helps in developing balanced and healthier relationships by filling mind, body and soul with an exuberant appreciation for life.

The breast reflexes

The breast reflexes (Figure 14.6) overlap the lung reflexes on the balls of the feet revealing the amount of loving care given and received, especially when growing up. The mammary glands are filled with 'memories' of the mothering process, or lack thereof, during these formative years. It may simply be a perception, belief or hearsay, yet it will still have a profound impact and affect one's expectations around nurturing. The actual size of the breasts, particularly on females, indicates how well equipped they feel in the giving of themselves emotionally, along with the amount of care they feel worthy of receiving. This can fluctuate enormously, according to innermost feelings of wellbeing or illness. A *breast cyst* can develop around accumulated sadness and emotional pain, which once acknowledged, makes it so much easier to relinquish these growths of discontent. Caress these reflexes (p. 255) for mind, body and soul to feel nurtured and make up for any perceived lack of care. The recipient can then feel better about themselves, regardless of what happened to them when they were a child.

Insight

The breast reflexes also reveal the capacity to love oneself and others. A newborn baby instinctively latches onto its mother's breasts, relying on this form of nourishment until weaned – that's the natural scenario. There is some concern that the increase in bottle-feeding could cause breast issues later on, either in the mother or their offspring.

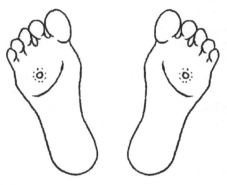

Figure 14.6 The breast reflexes.

The thymus gland

The thymus gland reflexes (Figure 14.7), on the inner edges, halfway down the balls of the feet, represent the 'seat of the soul'. They generally feel like tiny indentations on most feet but tend to be slightly swollen in the very young, as well as in the elderly

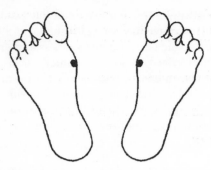

Figure 14.7 *The thymus gland reflexes.*

and during times of extreme vulnerability. The thymus gland steps in whenever feeling under attack or unfairly criticized; in fact any soul-destroying circumstances can adversely affect the thymus gland. When these reflexes *swell*, it's from trying to reach out for more space to be oneself and for personal recognition; whereas *hard skin* forms to act as a shield when concerned about feeling defenceless or helpless when constantly attacking oneself for not being good enough. The thymus gland reflexes sink from the utter exhaustion of having to constantly justify everything in an attempt to stop ongoing emotional abuse and endless criticism. *Bunions* appear when needing more space to 'just be' or when trying to break free from a stifling emotional environment that traps the soul and robs it of its individuality. When massaging the feet, spend extra time on these reflexes for any *thymus disorder*, to build up inner strength; for *AIDS*, to provide a relentless belief in one's uniqueness; for *bunions*, to free the soul of its many restraints; for *mastitis*, to alleviate the difficulty of having to meet so many emotional demands. Stimulating the thymus gland reflexes (p. 250) reconnects the recipient with their true spirit and makes the recipient proud to be an individual.

Insight

The thymus gland, the heart or love centre, is the 'seat of the soul'. It's extremely receptive to praise but exceptionally vulnerable to abuse, revealed by the build-up of hard skin over these reflexes. Bunions shove the thymus gland reflexes to the side due to inner turmoil and exaggerated feelings of self-doubt. Massaging the thymus gland reflexes helps to revitalize the true essence of the spirit.

Nothing is a threat, unless allowed to be.

The oesophagus

The oesophagus reflexes (Figure 14.8) extend from the mouth reflexes, along the inner edges of the big toe necks and balls of the feet, to the start of the insteps, revealing the courage to follow through with personal decisions. Their appearances are influenced by whatever is uppermost in the mind, as well as feelings towards what is being taken in, or shoved down the throat, on a daily basis. A ridge of *hard skin* appears over these reflexes when life is really difficult to swallow or when concealing the frustration of having been 'taken in'; they turn *white*, when tired of having things 'thrust down the gullet'; *red*, from anger, frustration or embarrassment at having to ingest unpalatable situations; occasionally they turn *blue* from the hurt of being taken advantage of; *flaky skin* indicates extreme irritability at becoming involved, despite being unsure of what's going on. Massaging the oesphagus reflexes (p. 262) clears the way for the recipient to move ahead with certainty and with the relief of knowing that they are back on track.

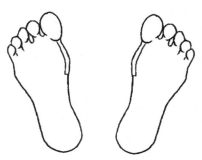

Figure 14.8 The oesophagus reflexes.

> **Insight**
> When life becomes hard to swallow, the oesophagus reflexes
> are the first to complain. Surrounded by overwhelming
> emotions, they become constrained and restricted, which only
> compounds the issue. Reflexology makes it easier to take in
> new life experiences, as well as any uncertainty, which makes
> life far more palatable.

The airways

The airway reflexes (Figure 14.9) extend from the bases of the big
toes to approximately halfway down the inner edges of the balls of
the feet, partially overlapping the oesophagus reflexes. Massaging
these reflexes enhances the exchange of vital life force energies and
opens the recipient up to all kinds of incredible possibilities.

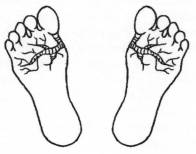

Figure 14.9 The airway reflexes.

The elbows

The elbow reflexes (Figure 14.10) are usually really noticeable
on the feet because they tend to stick out halfway down the outer
edges, showing just how much 'elbow room' is needed to be oneself.

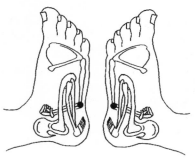

Figure 14.10 The elbow reflexes.

The knees

The primary reflexes for the knees (Figure 14.11) are situated in the middle of the balls of the feet, over the nipple reflexes, whereas their secondary reflexes (Figure 14.12) are on the outer edges of the feet, between the shoulder and elbow reflexes. The knees provide incredible flexibility when it comes to moving ahead. By bending to accommodate any adjustments, they expand possibilities. Knee disorders generally indicate that things are 'not in order' making it hard to give in or adapt to any unwelcome changes or differences of opinion. Kneading these reflexes helps the recipient to turn the corner with greater understanding and more compassion.

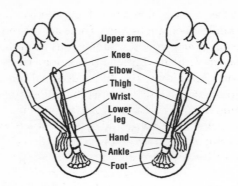

Figure 14.11 The primary knee reflexes.

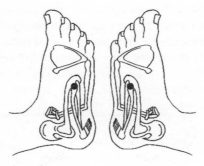

Figure 14.12 The secondary knee reflexes.

> ### Insight
>
> Knees instinctively bend for progress to be made so that
> mind and body can move easily through life. Their flexibility
> reveals the ability to take action or stand still when required.
> Massaging these reflexes encourages greater adaptability to
> the ups and downs of life.

The solar plexus

The solar plexus reflexes (Figure 14.13) extend from the inner
edges of the insteps to the central hollows immediately beneath

the balls of the feet, although, in reflexology, you will be accessing them via the middle indentations only. These are the most powerful reflexes on the feet; they induce instantaneous calm that spreads throughout the whole being during a reflexology treatment.

The solar plexus is also known as the 'abdominal brain' and, as such, is favourably or adversely affected by deep-seated feelings about everything that's happening or not happening. This is the gut feel of whether something should be done or left well alone, as well as who and what to get involved with. Too much or too little emotion really upsets the solar plexus, causing its reflexes to either *sink* from emotional exhaustion or *swell* from being completely overwhelmed. *Lines* on these reflexes are indicative of inner turmoil or feeling emotionally pulled apart. Reflexology soothes any uncertainty and reduces extreme sensitivity so that the recipient is less likely to overreact to distressing, nerve-racking situations. Instead they can discover an inner knowing of what to do with an innate understanding that everything is exactly as it should be.

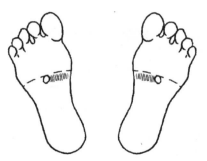

Figure 14.13 *The solar plexus reflexes.*

Insight

The solar plexus reflexes are the most highly charged and powerful on the feet. They are exceptionally useful for reassuring, calming, soothing and centring. With such strong astrological and symbolic connections between the feet and the solar plexus, each ganglion represents the five virtues of kindness, justice, love, wisdom and truth.

The ribs

The reflexes for the ribcage (Figure 14.14) cover a fair size of the balls on the feet before expanding around the outer edges and onto the tops, opposite the balls of the feet. These reflect the capacity to emotionally reinforce and back one's true feelings on the side, as well as in the background, since this is where the more unmanageable emotions reside. These reflexes complain when 'getting it in the ribs' or when there's a 'thorn in the side'. Meanwhile the ligaments on the tops of the feet can become taut from the strain of seeking additional emotional strength during particularly challenging times. Furthermore the upper surfaces become puffy when there's a buildup of unshed tears that are repeatedly shoved into the background. Massaging these reflexes provides the poignant strength and resourcefulness required to get through emotionally fraught times.

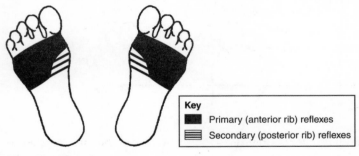

Key
■■ Primary (anterior rib) reflexes
≡ Secondary (posterior rib) reflexes

Figure 14.14 The ribcage reflexes.

Insight

The tops of the feet reflect the back and the past. This is where long lost memories are tucked away and unresolved issues or feelings are dumped to dissipate into the unconscious. Tight, prominent tendons appear here when holding back or putting up a huge resistance, whereas puffiness can be due to hanging on to unshed tears.

The lower arms

The lower arm reflexes (Figure 14.15) extend from the elbow reflexes to the wrist reflexes on the outer edges of both feet, symbolizing the ability to reach out and assist mind, body and soul through life. Their lower sections are affected by feelings, while their upper halves are influenced by the impetus to act and react.

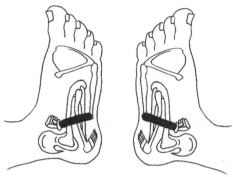

Figure 14.15 The lower arm reflexes.

The shins

The shin reflexes (Figure 14.16) extend from the knee reflexes to the feet reflexes on the outer edges of both feet, as well as on the soles. Their lower portions are subjected to the impact of emotions, whereas their upper sections are influenced by the body's actions and reactions to moving ahead.

Insight

Bunions are a sign of feeling out of place! Taking the thymus gland, the 'seat of soul', with them, only compounds the issue. Encourage the big toes to stand up for themselves, using any digit to straighten them, to boost emotional strength.

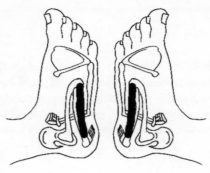

Figure 14.16 The shin reflexes.

The upper thoracic vertebrae

The upper thoracic vertebrae, which form the upper spine, are
reflected (Figure 14.17) along the bony ridges on the inner edges
of the balls of both feet, revealing the amount of emotional support
received. When under a lot of pressure or during really distressing
times, these bony ridges may give in and appear to *collapse*, especially
when there's little or no emotional encouragement; whereas they
bulge unmercifully whenever reaching out for additional strength
to get through a particularly challenging period. Soothing these
reflexes eases the discomfort of feeling bewildered and encourages
the recipient to be less critical of themselves and others.

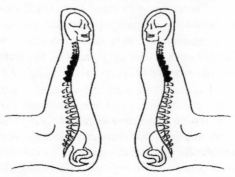

Figure 14.17 The upper back reflexes.

Liberating the breath

Massaging the balls of the feet is a great way of setting the spirit free, making it so much easier to breathe! With the breath liberated there is less tension in the ribcage, allowing the lungs to expand more fully, which means that any trapped emotions can now escape. With less frustration, bewilderment and fear, an enormous weight is lifted off the chest and the sense of relief is so great that the recipient is totally invigorated.

> If you wish for kindness, be kind to yourself,
> If you yearn for the truth, be true to yourself,
> For what you give of yourself is always reflected back.

The heart

The heart reflexes (Figure 14.18), on the inside edges where the balls of the feet and the insteps meet, are larger on the left foot because of the way in which the heart is angled. Positioned between the feeling area and the active parts of the body makes it possible to 'Do everything with heart and soul!' It's the centre of love and joy and loves nourishing and caring for all the body's needs but, to do this, it relies on the complete acceptance of oneself and others. Distressing situations 'tear at the heart' causing these reflexes to either *enlarge* when plagued by emotional issues or when reaching out for more love and affection; *fade* or *sink*, from having opened up but receiving precious little, if anything, in return; minuscule *blood blisters* sometimes appear over these reflexes from a 'bleeding heart'; *hard skin* forms as a protective shield against any further emotional damage; a *cut*, immediately beneath the heart reflexes, can appear when feeling 'cut off' or 'cut up' after a traumatic event, such as a divorce, separation or death. Caressing the heart reflexes encourages gushes of love to infiltrate the mind and body, as well as rekindle the spirit, so that the gift of life is once again fully appreciated!

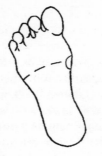
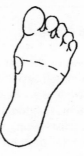

Figure 14.18 The heart reflexes.

Insight

A physically healthy heart is an emotionally happy heart. Finding love, joy and fulfilment in life ensures the flow of positive energies throughout the body.

The blood and circulation

The blood circulates, from the heart, around the whole body, distributing love and joy to each and every cell, which is enhanced when happy and relaxed. Constant despondency, however, really upsets the heart and can interfere not only with the blood flow, but its composition as well. This can, in time, increase the possibility of heart and circulatory diseases. Heart failure, from feeling a failure, makes it particularly difficult to circulate due to the disastrous lack of self-confidence.

When massaging the feet, give additional attention to the heart reflexes for all cardiac and blood disorders, so that inner harmony can be reinstated, along with an unimpeded flow of love and joy throughout; also for *anaemia*, to re-establish inner strength by boosting self-worth; for *arteriosclerosis*, to release pressure on the arteries; for *bleeding*, to replace deep sadness with greater understanding; for *high blood pressure*, to resolve disturbing emotional issues so that the blood vessels can expand and embrace new beginnings; for *low blood pressure*, to re-establish the gush of happiness to encourage self-acceptance; for *blood clotting* and *cholesterol* issues, to open up the channels of communication so that they remain viable; for *heartburn*, to release the gripping fear of heart-rending issues; for *blood acidity*, to neutralize bitterness and replace it with an appreciation for the good things in life; for *increased white blood cells*, to naturally fortify the whole body when there is perceived abuse, mentally, emotionally or physically; for *leukaemia*, to release unexpressed resentment at the heartlessness of it all; and for *varicose veins*, to strip out and discard disagreeable and discouraging circumstances. Reflexology re-establishes the flow of blood by giving the recipient a renewed passion for life.

Circulation is life, stagnation is death.

10 QUESTIONS TO CONSIDER

1 Where do emotions come from?

2 Which major systems and organs are connected to feelings about yourself and others?

3 Where are the eye reflexes and why are they so important?

4 What is intuition? How intuitive are you? What can be done to enhance intuition?

5 Which reflexes are mirrored onto the balls of both feet?

6 What do the changing colours on the feet mean?

7 What do the chest and breast reflexes reveal?

8 What effect does massaging the thymus gland reflexes have?

9 Why are the solar plexus reflexes believed to be the most powerful points on the feet?

10 Where are the heart reflexes? What can affect the circulation of blood?

10 THINGS TO REMEMBER

1   The second 'feeling' toes are connected to the respiratory and circulatory systems, as well as the heart, revealing emotions, along with feelings, sense of self-worth and self-esteem.

2   The second toes and balls of the feet resonate to the colours green and pink, and also to the element of air.

3   The eyes, linked to the second toes, are the 'windows to the soul', with whatever is being seen bringing up emotion.

4   Massaging the eye reflexes also stimulates the pineal gland, which brings light to situations, balancing the body's cycles.

5   Lungs represent the ability to take in life for the realization of one's full potential.

6   Massaging the thymus gland reflexes, halfway down the inner edges on the balls of the feet, boosts the immune system and counteracts feelings of vulnerability.

7   The solar plexus is the abdominal or feeling brain, so massaging its reflexes, which are the slight indentations just underneath the centre of the balls of the feet, instantly calms mind, body and soul.

8   Massaging the balls of the feet liberates the breath by easing any tension in the ribcage, so that the lungs can expand and trapped emotions can be released.

9   Massaging the heart reflexes, on the inside edges of the balls of the feet, helps to heal heart-breaking emotions.

10 Blood circulating from the heart distributes uppermost emotions, so massaging the heart reflexes encourages a free flow of blood and a renewed passion for life.

15

The third toes and upper halves
of the insteps

In this chapter you will learn:
- *about the impact of actions and reactions*
- *about the role of food*
- *about things that influence digestion.*

The third 'doing' toes

The third toes (Figure 15.1) are known as the 'doing toes',
revealing all that is in mind when it comes to taking action, or
how to react to what's going on. The impact of what is done
or not done then shows up on the upper halves of the sole insteps.
The third toes are energetically connected to the middle fingers,
as well as the cheeks, ears, nose, top halves of the lower arms and
lower shins, and the upper abdomen. Their energy comes from
past experiences, the memories of which accumulate in the
liver. The other parts of the body that are also involved are the
duodenum, pancreas, stomach, spleen and adrenal glands, all of
which influence the actions of the upper digestive tract and its
related parts.

The element that works in their favour is fire, which is both
destructive and constructive by its nature, symbolizing the need to
get rid of the old before starting something new, while the colour

to which they resonate is yellow, the colour of intelligence and inspiration.

Concentrate on massaging the third toes and upper halves of the insteps for *influenza*, to flush out infuriating irritabilities; for *abscesses*, to drain away deep hurts; for *body odour*, to boost confidence; for *middle back problems*, to replace guilt, 'tucked in the small of the back', with wisdom gained from life's experiences. Reflexology encourages the third toes to stand up for themselves. Better still, it encourages the recipient to repeatedly run all their brilliant ideas through their system, in the hope that they do something really worthwhile with them and, in so doing, rediscover just how substantial and resourceful they really are.

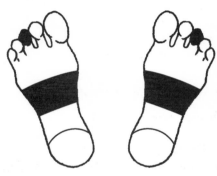

Figure 15.1 The third toes and their related parts.

Insight

Do something that has been put off for some time – it's such a relief! Do something fearful – it dissipates the fear! Doing what you love, means never having to work another day.

The nose

The nose, with its reflexes halfway along the inner edges of each toe (Figure 15.2), takes in air to keep mind, body and soul alive and alert. It also detects smells, which are the most evocative of all the senses. By 'following the nose' it's possible to stay on track since each whiff can be inextricably linked to a specific memory, be it a situation, person or event. The mere thought of this memory can have the power to 'turn the nose up' in disgust, or bring a smile to the face. The appearance of the nose, its size, shape and colour, is affected by the acknowledgement of whatever is achieved so that the nose can be held high with dignity and pride (but not too much because that leads to snobbery!). For ongoing success it's best to keep 'the nose out of other people's business', and not be too 'nosy'. On the other hand, 'paying through the nose' could put 'the nose out of joint'. Reflexology heightens the recipient's sense of smell so that they can stay on track and achieve all that they came to do.

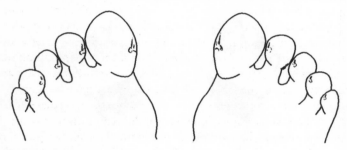

Figure 15.2 The nose reflexes.

When things 'get up the nose' it's usually because of being a perfectionist, who gets highly irritated by the way others do or don't do things, especially when they 'block the way'. Massaging the nose reflexes ensures greater tolerance, so that things can settle down long enough for the 'air to clear' and for the approach to life to change. Rub these reflexes (p. 228) well for all *nasal disorders*, to instil greater understanding and leniency, so that the focus is directed onto what's important; for *adenoid disorders*, to reduce irritability at not having 'the space to breathe'; and for *colds*, to unleash a mass of exasperating circumstances that have 'got up the nose', making the way clear for new beginnings. Massaging the nose reflexes helps the recipient to recognize what a truly amazing individual they are, what they've achieved in life for the betterment of themselves and others.

The ears

The ear reflexes (Figure 15.3), midway along the outer edges of
the toes, represent the capacity to hear and really listen to what is
going on or not going on. They have an inborn ability to transform
sound waves into meaningful message that give direction, guidance
and balance, especially from the inner voice. Problems arise when
things 'go in one ear and out the other' or if they keep 'falling on
deaf ears', which generally happens when constantly receiving an
'earful'. Massaging these reflexes (p. 229) opens the ears. Give
additional attention to these reflexes for *deafness*, to replace fearful
sounds and conversations of the past with greater discernment;
for *earache*, to ease the pain of hurtful comments, either voiced or
muttered 'beneath the breath'; or for *loss of balance*, to centre the
mind so that both sides are given a fair hearing. Reflexology helps
the recipient to pick up and concentrate on what's important so
that they can move ahead with the sound knowledge of who and
what they are.

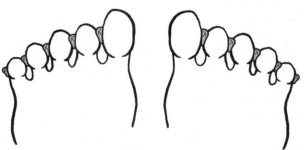

Figure 15.3 The ear reflexes.

The cheeks

The cheek reflexes (Figure 15.4) are the small bulges, just off-centre, towards the outer edges of all the toes, revealing the degree of confidence when it comes to being 'cheeky' and doing something that others might consider impudent. Rub these reflexes well to treat apathy and instil enthusiasm as well as re-establish a purpose in life. Give them extra attention for *meningitis*, so that the anger and frustration of ideas being held back can be replaced with the determination to share unique and unusual ideas, regardless of the consequences. Reflexology encourages the recipient to do what they really need to do, even when others try to stop them from being so different.

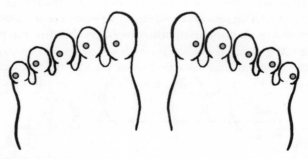

Figure 15.4 The cheek reflexes.

The digestive process

The *digestive process* is immediately affected by change, particularly a change of mind or heart. Discomfort comes from fluctuating emotions that range from extreme ecstasy to intense anger, from incredible fear to unconstrained excitement, or from severe nervousness to unbelievable confidence. Detrimental reactions from others about what has or hasn't happened can cause extreme tension throughout the digestive tract, upsetting the harmonious expansion and contraction of the alimentary canal, which, in turn, hampers the progress of food. The resultant irritability and increased acidity come from a build-up of resentment and bitterness, which then alter the chemical composition and disturb metabolism. Over time, extra layers of fat may develop to act as shock absorbers or to prevent further emotional damage from harmful psychological attacks. Any of this can show up in the upper halves of the insteps, with *wrinkles* highlighting concern and *lines* revealing tight restraints, deep commitments or feeling tied or caught up. Reflexology helps the recipient to deal with adversity and encourages them to use it as an opportunity to get to know themselves better.

Insight

The digestive system is one of the most extensive systems of the body, running from head to tail. Feelings invariably determine the intake of food, which is why intense emotions affect digestion. Fear loosens the bowels, whilst being tightly in control brings on constipation. Relax and go with the flow!

The liver

The liver is reflected (Figure 15.5) onto the triangular mound that occupies the bulk of the outer half of the right sole instep, along with a much smaller triangular area on the upper, inner quadrant of the left instep. Together they display the liver's lively characteristics, which are many, being the largest and most versatile organ in the body. Its multitude of vital functions are essential for keeping mind, body and soul well energized and active at all times; even though the bulk of its activities take place during sleep. The liver 'takes the brunt' whenever there's a build-up of frustration and anger, especially about something that happened or didn't happen in the past. Its reflexes become *distended* with needless resentment, or *sink* from utter exasperation, especially when pressured into meeting ludicrous social and family expectations. Kneading these reflexes (p. 258) keeps the liver in a harmonious state, first by ridding the body of toxic thoughts and noxious emotions, then by storing enthusiasm, coming from the satisfaction of things well done. The rejuvenated blood then infuses the whole with passion. The liver constantly draws on the energy of past events to fuel the present and ensure that something really worthwhile is achieved through having a life. At the same time, it generates sufficient heat to keep the body comfortable.

The liver is truly remarkable!

Insight

A clean liver is vital for the body to heal itself, which is why this energetic organ constantly strives to evict toxic thoughts and noxious memories. It can then infuse the blood with energy to be distributed throughout. Reflexology assists in the transformation of suppressed anger into a passion for life.

The liver gets really agitated when feeling absolutely 'livid', taking on and containing the bulk of inner fury, profound dissatisfaction and suppressed guilt. This is then likely to erupt from time to time, causing aggressiveness, extreme criticism and a foul temper. Massaging these reflexes (p. 258) assists in working through the past, transforming whatever happened into an asset, rather than a drawback. Spend extra time palpating the liver reflexes for *burns*, to release the intense desire to retaliate; for *chills*, to prevent the temptation to withdraw; for *colds*, to flush out irritating notions for a different perspective; for *fatigue*, to fill the whole with an enthusiasm for life that defies boredom and tiredness; for *fever*, to encourage heated emotions to surface and then dissipate; for *infection* and *inflammation*, to 'put out the fire' raging within; for *boils*, to bring to a head all those frustrations, that simmer beneath the skin, so that they burst and are done with; for *alcoholism*, to eliminate the need to drown sorrows by boosting self-acceptance; for *hepatitis*, for greater understanding of what went on in the past; as well as for *jaundice*, to change jaundiced outlooks. Reflexology assists the recipient in realizing that everything that happens is exactly as it should be, and is an opportunity to discover the truth about themselves and others.

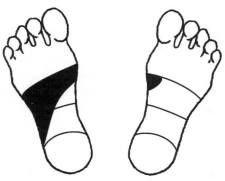

Figure 15.5 The liver reflexes.

The gall bladder

The tiny rounded swelling of the gall bladder reflex (Figure 15.6), towards the centre of the right sole instep, highlights the joy or animosity of all that happened, or didn't happen, in the past. A build up of resentment makes the bile bitter, which could explain the increase in gall bladder problems in the offspring of those who reluctantly participated in battle, due to the lingering memory of atrocities witnessed. The gall bladder reflex may *harden* when filled with bitter memories, so wheedle this reflex (p. 259) to coax out any hostility and replace it with forgiveness for themselves and others.

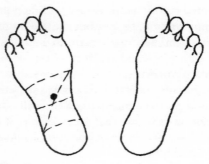

Figure 15.6 The gall bladder reflex.

Insight

The attitude of all organs originates in the gall bladder since it rules decisions. Angry behaviour and rash decisions, from excessive bile, stem from resentment, while indecisiveness and timidity are signs of disharmony and weakness. Massaging the gall bladder reflex encourages greater understanding and ultimate forgiveness.

Forgiveness can't change the past but it can change the future.

The pancreas

Just above the 'waistline' of the feet, are the pancreatic reflexes (Figure 15.7), which extend from the centres of the sole insteps to the inner edges, revealing the satisfaction and pleasure derived from all activities, invariably based on the type of reaction and responses received from others. Problems generally show up in the body 18 months to two years after a traumatic event, although they can often be detected on the feet long before this. The pancreas gets upset when resentment gets in the way of enjoying life to the full because of not getting over what previously happened, be it a death, divorce, miscarriage, job loss, devastating move, serious accident and so on. Its reflexes *bulge* when reaching out for sympathy or requiring greater fulfilment and become quite *deflated* from the exhaustion of continually trying to please others to the detriment of oneself. Soothe the pancreatic reflexes (p. 259) when life has become too overwhelming and give them additional attention for *diabetes*, for past unhappiness to be put into perspective; *hypoglycaemia*, for renewed enthusiasm and greater appreciation; as well as for *pancreatitis*, to ensure that everything is done with absolute pleasure. Reflexology makes sure that the recipient's spirit is well replenished, to the delight and complete satisfaction of their whole being.

Insight

The pancreas derives its energy from feelings about events that occurred or were missed. For the ideal balance, it helps if the events of the past are understood and honoured in a favourable and loving manner.

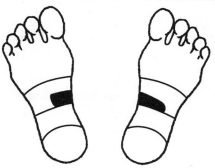

Figure 15.7 The pancreatic reflexes.

The spleen

The spleen ensures that everything is done with the appropriate amount of precision and attention to detail, according to family and social expectations. Its reflex is a small mound (Figure 15.8) on the upper outer quadrant of the left sole instep. It's likely to *enlarge* whenever there's an obsession or obsessive tendencies, particularly filled with outrage and revenge towards the family or society, and it *sinks* when tired of abiding by strict rules that seem so pointless. Palpate this reflex (p. 260) to bring out the very best in the recipient so that they are more tolerant of family members and society. Also give it additional attention for *arthritis*, for greater give and take within all that is done or not done; for *addictions*, to remove the compulsion to self-destruct and to rebuild a healthier self-image; for *unhealthy appetites*, for a more balanced approach in trying to please others; for *bulimia*, so life's opportunities can be taken in without feeling overwhelmed or inadequate; for *obesity*, to assist in resolving weighty issues; for *cellulite*, to stop self-criticism and promote greater belief in oneself; for *constipation*, to release burdensome beliefs that get in the way; for *diarrhoea*, to bring to a halt the need to run away; and for *haemorrhoids*, to no longer feel encumbered, strained or suppressed. Reflexology gives the recipient the faith to believe in all that they do so that, in the process, they gain greater appreciation for those around them.

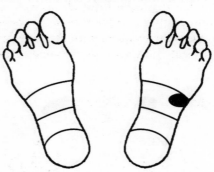

Figure 15.8 The spleen reflex.

Insight

The spleen, considered to be the body's clock, is a warehouse and depot for white and red blood cells that constantly filter worn out and hurt emotions. Being so closely linked to the mouth and lips, any critical and obsessive words or expressions can immediately upset it, especially when going out of the way to keep everybody happy.

The adrenal glands

The adrenal gland reflexes (Figure 15.9) are immediately beneath those of the solar plexus, with the right reflex being slightly lower and a little more central than that of the left. These glands provide incredible courage and resourcefulness for unique and innovative ideas to be put into practice, even though the way-out and unusual concepts may initially attract disapproval, adversity or criticism. These reflexes *swell* when feeling overcome by fear, anxiety or terror, or *sink* when defeated or lacking the courage of one's convictions or when feeling discouraged from constantly being under pressure to prove oneself. Stimulate these reflexes well (p. 251) for the audacity to do what has never been done before. Concentrate on them for any *adrenal disorder*, to boost inner strength and instil greater fortitude, as well as for *Addison's disease*, to encourage greater appreciation of personal assets. Reflexology provides the recipient with the determination to do things differently, just because everybody is different and unique!

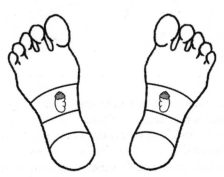

Figure 15.9 The adrenal gland reflexes.

Fear is emotionally, mentally, physically and spiritually taxing; it is also exceptionally disempowering. Fear feeds off fear, so focusing on it creates even more fear. The adrenal glands, with the helping hand of reflexology, assist in conquering fear and, instead, provide the courage to move ahead, even in the face of adversity.

The cardiac sphincter

The reflexes of the cardiac sphincter (Figure 15.10) are slight mounds that can be felt on the inner edges of both feet, where the balls of the feet meet the insteps. It's the muscular entrance to the stomach that lets food in but stops it from coming back again, that is until overwhelming emotions get the upper hand and cause nausea and vomiting. The build-up of heartfelt feelings can be enough to make anybody sick, causing *reflux* or *heartburn*. Reflexology makes stomaching life's events more manageable, no matter how scary or difficult they may at first seem.

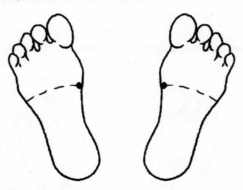

Figure 15.10 The cardiac sphincter reflexes.

Insight
The cardiac sphincter is the point of no return for food as it enters the stomach. Massaging these reflexes helps to calm

overwhelming emotions that are difficult to stomach. It also
assists in directing the food in the most beneficial way.

The stomach

The slightly bulbous stomach reflexes (Figure 15.11) cover the bulk
of the upper inner quadrant on the left sole instep, with a much
smaller triangular area on the corresponding part of the right sole
instep. They show just how well life is being 'stomached' or not,
and how events are being dealt with – all symbolized through food.
In fact, everything and anything that is done, or not done, is linked
to food; after all, food is what provides energy to get on and live
life. Furthermore, whatever things can or cannot be achieved, along
with whatever happens or doesn't happen, are highlighted by food,
be it through changes in appetite, the type of intake, the reaction to
food, or the likes and dislikes. The stomach is easily upset by the
unexpected, ongoing inactivity, a deep dread, extreme concern, or
a fear of taking on something new or unusual. Palpate these reflexes
well whenever anything disturbs the stomach, especially when unable
to 'stomach' what's going on; also for *abdominal cramps*, to release
the stomach from the gripping clutches of fear; for *vomiting*, to make
repulsive situations and circumstances more digestible; as well as
for *peptic ulcers*, to stop the gnawing feelings of something eating
away at the insides. Reflexology makes sure that sickness is seen
as an opportunity to become stronger, giving the recipient the guts
to deal with anything new or unexpected. It restores the recipient's
faith in their own capabilities.

When the body is sick and tired of all the moans and groans,
it will start playing up.

Insight

Sick to the stomach? Why? Perhaps it's all those upset
feelings about what was done or not done? After all, this is

(Contd)

where unresolved issues, especially those revolving around the mother, simmer. Massaging these reflexes soothes things over, putting them into a more manageable perspective.

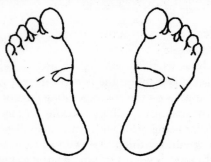

Figure 15.11 The stomach reflexes.

The pyloric sphincter

The pyloric sphincter reflex (Figure 15.12) feels like a minuscule ball, just under the ball of the right foot, in line with the join between the second and big toes. This muscular outlet of the stomach is greatly influenced by the ability to process all that is being taken in to be dealt with, depending on what happened in the past. Fear causes the pyloric sphincter to contract, which can lead to *pyloric stenosis*; more common in male babies, possibly because

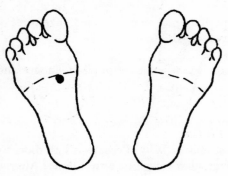

Figure 15.12 Pyloric sphincter reflex.

of being linked to the mother's unpalatable experiences with men, the thought of which still makes her sick. Soothing these reflexes provides the recipient with the reassurance that it's okay to move on regardless of what happened previously.

> Individuals become successful the moment they start moving towards a worthwhile goal.

The duodenum

The C-shape of the duodenum reflex (Figure 15.13) follows the perimeter of the upper inner quadrant of the right sole instep, revealing how past experiences are affecting the current situation in moving ahead. The gall bladder and pancreas fill the duodenum with the remnants of the past to assist in processing everyday events using the wisdom and confidence that can be attained when dealing with life. Massaging this reflex (p. 264) helps the recipient in using the past as an asset in the present.

> Experience is a hard teacher; it tests first and teaches later.

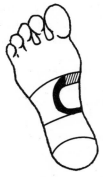
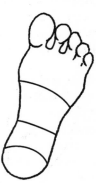

Figure 15.13 The duodenum reflex.

The jejunum

The jejunum reflex (Figure 15.14) extends along, or just above, the waistline mainly on the left foot, and is the connection between the duodenum and small intestine reflexes. It is affected by the amount of confidence in moving on to the next stage in the process of life. Soothing this reflex encourages the recipient to keep going, rather than give up midway.

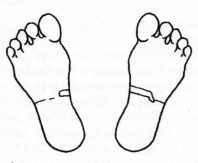

Figure 15.14 The jejunum reflex.

It's necessary to go inwards, to keep going outwards.

The middle back

The middle back reflexes (Figure 15.15) are reflected over the tops and insides of the upper halves of both insteps. Their appearance is influenced by the backing and support given to oneself in all that occurs or doesn't occur. It also mirrors any tasks or projects that the 'back has been turned on' and shows whether there's been a need to 'bend over backwards' to please others. A *prominent bone* may pop up on top of the foot, from time to time, when feeling pressured into getting things done; while *veins* frequently appear over this area, to reveal the unhappiness of the past or disclose what's going on in the background, which, thankfully, is being worked through to be got rid of once and for all.

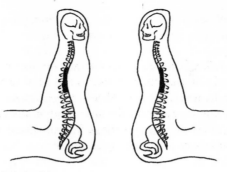

Figure 15.15 The middle back reflexes.

Doing what has always been done means that the results will always be the same!

Getting on with life

There are many advantages to modern technology, especially the drudgery that is taken out of mundane tasks that once took up huge chunks of time. There is now a chance to get on with developing creative talents. If, however, these opportunities are ignored or misused or wasted, then the additional time available is lost, which can be quite sickening. All the self-flagellating mind-talk is really upsetting, especially since the body is more than aware of what it's capable of doing, so it draws attention to this through specific symptoms; these effectively highlight deep dissatisfaction, extreme frustration or intense bewilderment, in the hope that something is done.

Yet, it's not just about getting on and doing something; it's more about the spirit with which it's done that makes the difference. Life on earth is all about taking an active role, living in the moment and focusing on what needs to be done for the betterment of all. Doing this is so empowering since it expands the level of self-awareness. There's not enough time to worry about what others are up to; they are entitled to live life their own way and hopefully they and many others benefit; otherwise it's up to them to deal with the consequences. Reflexology assists the recipient in being more considerate and aware of what they are doing, knowing that whatever is put out there has an uncanny knack of bouncing back!

Insight

Life can only change for the better when the appropriate steps are taken. Reflexology offers that extra boost of confidence and courage to be different!

Live well for today, for yesterday is but a dream and tomorrow a vision; today well lived, makes every yesterday a dream of happiness and every tomorrow a vision of hope.

10 QUESTIONS TO CONSIDER

1   Which thoughts influence the condition of the third toes?

2   What parts of the body are these toes connected to?

3   Where are the nose, ear and cheek reflexes? Why do they play up from time to time?

4   What types of input detrimentally affect the digestive tract?

5   When do the liver and gall bladder reflexes change their appearance?

6   What is toxic to the body?

7   With so much diabetes and hypoglycaemia around, how can massaging the pancreatic and splenic reflexes assist in making the improvements needed?

8   Are the right and left adrenal gland reflexes in the same position? If not, how do they differ? What's their role in determining what's done or not done?

9   What affects the stomach, cardiac and pyloric sphincter reflexes, and how can massaging these reflexes influence the digestive process?

10 Where are the middle back reflexes? What causes them to change their appearance?

10 THINGS TO REMEMBER

1 *The third toes represent what is done or not done with one's own ideas.*

2 *The upper halves of the sole insteps contain the upper digestive reflexes, namely the liver, gall bladder, duodenum, stomach, pancreas, spleen and adrenal glands.*

3 *The third toes and upper halves of the sole insteps resonate to the colour yellow and the element of fire.*

4 *The nose, ears and cheek reflexes also reflect actions and reactions to life experiences.*

5 *The digestive process is affected by thoughts and changing emotions, as well as by other people's actions and reactions.*

6 *Massaging the liver reflexes, on the upper triangular area of the right sole instep, helps to release toxic thoughts and noxious emotions, re-energizing the whole.*

7 *Stimulating the pancreatic reflexes, just above the waistline of both feet, boosts the amount of satisfaction, pleasure and happiness derived from one's actions.*

8 *Massaging the splenetic reflex, on the upper outer quadrant of the left sole instep, deals with the extremes of obsessive or apathetic behaviour, restoring the balance in getting things done.*

9 *Kneading the adrenal gland reflexes, immediately beneath the solar plexus reflexes on both feet, with the right reflex being slightly lower and more central than the left, provides the courage to be innovative and different, especially in the face of adversity.*

10 *Soothing the stomach reflexes, mainly in the upper inner quadrant of the left sole instep, helps in stomaching and dealing with life.*

16

The fourth toes and lower portions of the insteps

In this chapter you will learn:
- *the importance of relationships*
- *how to attain a balance*
- *the need to be more discerning.*

The fourth 'relationship' toes

The fourth toes are the 'communication and relationship toes' that show how well individuals relate to who and what they are, as well as to others. This has a direct or indirect impact on the way in which they communicate, the impact of which is then mirrored onto the lower halves of both sole insteps, where the bulk of the lower digestive tract reflexes are situated. These include the small intestine, appendix and large colon, part of the excretory system reflexes (specifically the kidneys) plus some of the female reproductive system reflexes (namely the fallopian tubes and ovaries). Incidentally, the energy of the ovaries is present in both genders. Then on the tops of the feet, directly opposite the lower halves of the insteps, are the lower middle back reflexes, as well as the secondary access to all the above organs and glands.

The fourth toes are energetically linked to the mouth, ring fingers, bottom halves of the upper arms and thighs, as well as the lower abdomen. The element that unites them is water, which ensures a good 'flow of conversation', and soothes things over when 'waves are being made'. Too much water causes *oedema*, a sign of 'drowning' in the wake of overwhelming emotions while, conversely, the body 'dries up' and becomes *dehydrated* when giving too much of oneself to others. The colour that relates well to these parts is orange, a wonderful mixture of yellow and red that brings the vibrancy out in everything and everyone. Relationships create an awareness of the abundant joy and happiness that can be gained from all interactions, both internally and externally.

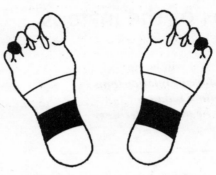

Figure 16.1 The fourth toes and related reflexes.

The mouth

Whatever is said, be it mentally or aloud, has an immediate impact on all concerned. Words are so powerful that they can make or break a relationship. The energy of the unspoken word stays in the mouth, affecting everything that passes through it, as it enters or leaves the body. This energy also influences eating, as well as the air being breathed, along with the words that pass through the lips. The mouth, meanwhile, serves as an essential link between the inner and outer worlds, with the nature of these interactions having a profound, negative or positive, effect, which then influences the body's chemical make-up.

On an energetic level, everybody is like a magnet, intentionally, but not necessarily consciously, attracting into their lives those individuals and circumstances that best mirror what's going on at a much deeper level. This highlights the beliefs and memories being clung to, usually subconsciously, and their influence on the production of all bodily fluids, particularly the digestive juices. The efficiency of these is also greatly influenced by the amount of give and take within relationships. Each change of mind changes the characteristics of the mouth, either fractionally or quite noticeably. These reflexes *sink* when tired of the same old thing being said over and over again or *swell* when wanting to 'speak up' and say what's on the mind. The mouth, teeth, tongue and gums are all bunched together on two minuscule reflexes, approximately two thirds of the way down the inner edges of each toe (Figure 16.2). They reflect the influence, good and bad, that decisions have on the rest of the body, as they reverberate throughout the whole. Whatever is communicated and relayed affects every cell to some extent or other, which is then picked up and reflected onto the lower halves of both sole insteps.

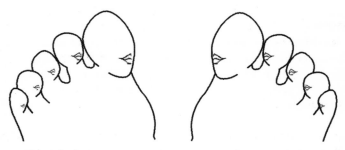

Figure 16.2 *The mouth reflexes.*

When opening the mouth, it's best not to put a foot into it!

Insight

The mouth takes in new ideas and provides nourishment for the whole. Problems arise when set opinions, a closed mind, the inability to take in new ideas or keeping the mouth shut get in the way. So look out for patches of hard skin over the mouth reflexes.

Spend extra time massaging the mouth reflexes (p. 261) for any mouth disorders, such as *halitosis*, to replace festering words with greater understanding; for *bleeding gums*, to restore confidence in the decisions made; for *cerebral palsy*, for a more lively exchange of energy, no matter how bad things may appear to be; for *cold sores*, to bring some warmth into conversations; for *epilepsy*, to prevent 'throwing a fit' or 'biting the tongue' when there's a misunderstanding or being misunderstood; for *gum disorders*, for the confidence to make up one's own mind; for *neuralgia*, to ease the anguish of rejection or ridicule when 'speaking out of turn'; for *strokes*, to bring to an end the self-inflicted pressure of trying to meet unrealistically high expectations; for *stuttering*, to boost confidence in sharing unbelievable ideas; for *tooth problems*, to take away the agony and pain of decision making; and for *tinnitus*, to alert the mind to messages from the inner voice. Massaging these reflexes helps the recipient speak up and share their truth, without necessarily agreeing and without fear of what others might have to say on the matter.

Insight

Skin that has a rippled appearance, on the lower insteps, indicates the many ups and downs within relationships. Simultaneously grab the big toe and little toe on the right foot and gently raise the foot to help these dissipate. Repeat on the left foot.

Begin by telling the truth and never stop.

The small intestine

The small intestine is linked to the give and take within relationships and so it knows what's 'good' and should be 'taken on board' and what isn't so agreeable and should be left well alone. Its reflexes (Figure 16.3) occupy the bulk of the lower halves of both sole insteps highlighting the benefits that are constantly derived from ongoing interactions, symbolized by the intake and assimilation of food. The small intestine assists in absorbing new life force energies for ongoing growth within relationships since these refreshing energies are so very influential in the development of the new cells.

The small intestine reflexes *swell* when weighed down from taking on too much; *flatten* when feeling flat from giving too much of oneself, when fearful or lacking self-worth; become *dry* when deprived or drained; *wrinkle* when concerned; have *crossed lines* from being at a 'crossroads' or at 'cross purposes' or have a 'cross to bear' or just 'cross'; *netted lines* from feeling trapped, 'tied down' or 'caught up' in a relationship; deep *vertical lines* due to a division or cut-off point; *scattered lines* from internal chaos and havoc. The colours of the reflexes (see Chapter 8) reveal fluctuating moods and changing emotions.

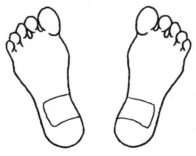

Figure 16.3 The small intestine reflexes.

Massaging the small intestine reflexes helps to create a much-needed balance in all relationships, internally and externally. Concentrate on these reflexes for *insect bites*, to prevent biting remarks or from feeling sucked dry; for *blisters*, to soothe any friction; for *candida*, to become more centred and less frustrated at being pulled in many directions, trying to please others; for *fever blisters*, to increase tolerance so that heated emotions don't cause friction; for *cysts*, to relax the need to hang on to a mass of hurts; for *fungi*, to discourage being taken advantage of and relentless memories from taking over; for *oedema*, to expel cumbersome beliefs that weigh on the mind, body and soul; for *parasites*, to evict those who energetically live off others; and for *malabsorption syndrome*, to replenish the whole through an improved intake of data and ideas. Reflexology facilitates the absorption of the beneficial aspects of life so that, by becoming wiser, the recipient knows how best to relate to others.

> Whatever role is being played in relationships, the game is always the same.

The ileo-caecal valve

The ileo-caecal valve reflex (Figure 16.4), on the outer corner of the right lower sole instep, represents the strong muscular connection between the small and large intestines. It facilitates the onward movement of anything that is no longer required in the body, so that no more time or energy is wasted. Massage this reflex (p. 267) well to bridge the gap between what was and what is still to come.

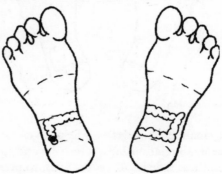

Figure 16.4 *The ileo-caecal valve reflexes.*

Insight
The ileo-caecal valve is the doorway between the small intestine and colon; it's the beginning of the letting go process of anything that is wasting time and energy. Massage it well to prevent any emotional backtracking.

The appendix

The finger-shaped appendix is considered by some to be surplus to human requirements. Its minuscule reflex (Figure 16.5) is just below the ileo-caecal valve reflex on the right foot only. The only time that the appendix grumbles is when in a dead-end relationship or when life is going nowhere in particular. The infuriation of being in such an awkward position can make the situation so bad that the appendix may even burst. Massage the appendix reflex well for *appendicitis,* to replace the frustration of being at the 'end of one's tether' with greater empathy. Reflexology helps the recipient let go of anything that no longer serves them.

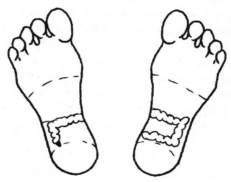

Figure 16.5 The appendix reflex.

Insight

Even if the appendix has been removed, its energy remains, so always massage this reflex to soothe the remnants of any emotional leftovers and frustrations regarding dead-end relationships.

The bowels

The reflexes of the large intestine (Figure 16.6), otherwise known as the colon, border most of the lower sole insteps. There are four main parts: the ascending colon reflex, stretching up the outer edge of the lower right sole instep; the transverse colon reflexes, extending across both feet, just beneath the waistlines, rising slightly as it reaches the outer edge of the left lower instep; the descending colon reflex, going down the outer edge of the lower left sole instep and finally the sigmoid colon reflex, following the boundary between the left instep and heel. The large intestine or colon contains remnants of the past, which, if left to loiter for too long needlessly bog down the mind, body and soul. Its reflex mirrors the innate need for all accomplishments to be recognized and acknowledged, which is why the transverse colon reflexes *swell*, when there's constant antagonism and competitiveness within, because of never being satisfied; or when pressured into performing better than one's best, usually for all the wrong reasons. Cajole the bowel reflexes to evacuate old thoughts and worn-out emotions that would otherwise waste time and sap the body of its energy. Extra attention needs to be given to these reflexes for colon disorders, to expel the dread of failure; for *colic* in babies, to pacify the mother's impatience; for *colitis*, to relieve the agony of constantly having to compete and beat the clock, along with being infuriated for being under constant pressure; and for *spastic colon*, to relieve the irritability of always having to be better than one's best, no matter what. Reflexology encourages the recipient to keep moving on for ongoing bowel movements; reminding them that a little bit of pressure, from time to time, can go a long way in creating more of an urge for success.

Insight

Coaxing the colon reflexes helps 'control freaks' to ease their tight grip on life, in the hope that they will let go of any wasteful thoughts and beliefs that keep getting in the way, so that they can just go with the flow!

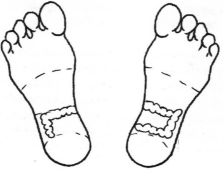

Figure 16.6 The large intestine/colon reflexes.

Life is not given to be wasted and ignored; it is given as a
blessing to be made the most of.

The female reproductive organs

Some female reproductive organs are reflected onto the soles, while
the remainder can be found on the inner heels. These reflexes reveal
how feminine attributes enhance personal relationships by adding
the soft touch. Massaging them creates a greater acceptance and
appreciation of the female role in the formation, accommodation
and nurturing of new beginnings.

The ovaries

The ovary reflexes (Figure 16.7), situated in the outer lower corner
of both sole insteps, reflect the ability to create and generate new
concepts, not just in the form of babies, but also in shaping and
developing ongoing ideas. These tiny reflexes feel like two minuscule
water bubbles situated just beneath the surface. When menstruating,
the reflex of the ovulating ovary enlarges, while that of the resting

ovary virtually disappears. The contraceptive pill prevents ovulation, making these minute reflexes barely discernible.

Swollen ovary reflexes usually indicate accumulated frustration, when bursting with novel notions but having no idea of what to do with them, while *sunken* reflexes generally indicate that amazing notions are being aborted, or there's possible conflict with another woman. Caress these reflexes (p. 252) to make sure that exciting new concepts are constantly generated to bring about much-needed changes in the world.

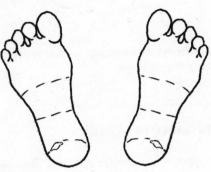

Figure 16.7 The ovary reflexes.

Insight

The ovaries contain ancestral knowledge, used to balance mind, body and soul. Their pro-creative abilities connect them to the source of creativity, which provides the soul with an opportunity to regenerate human energies.

The fallopian tubes

The primary reflexes for the fallopian tubes and their fingers (Figure 16.8) stretch across the soles, along or near the base of the fleshy sole instep, just above the heels, while their secondary reflexes (Figure 16.9) extend over the ankle creases from the one ankle bone to the other. The fallopian tubes make sure that new concepts have a chance of being fertilized so that they can come to life. Soothing these reflexes makes this a viable and worthwhile proposition.

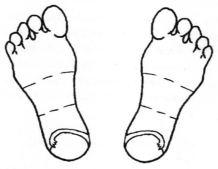

Figure 16.8 *The primary fallopian tube and finger reflexes.*

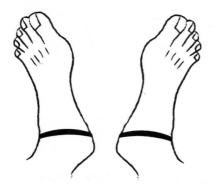

Figure 16.9 *The secondary fallopian tube and finger reflexes.*

The kidneys

The kidneys are involved in the initial process of letting go of worked-through thoughts and obsolete emotions that would otherwise overload the body and make it burst! Their reflexes (Figure 16.10) are tiny, kidney-shaped vertical mounds, on the lower sole instep areas, immediately beneath the adrenal gland reflexes, with the right reflex being slightly lower and a fraction further in, towards the centre of the right foot, than the left.

They *swell* to show that a stack of hefty thoughts and overpowering emotions are being worked through; they *harden* when filled with constant disappointments and disillusionment, and they *sink* when feeling betrayed, deflated or defeated. Milking these reflexes eases the process of letting go. Spend more time on them for *nephritis*, to eliminate the anger and frustration of being constantly thwarted, and for *childhood ailments*, to discourage parents from acting like kids. Reflexology helps in flushing away the past in the knowledge that life flows so much more easily when there's nothing in the way.

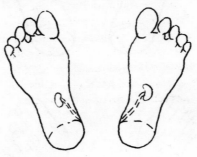

Figure 16.10 The kidney reflexes.

The ureter

The ureter reflexes (Figure 16.11) extend from the mid-point of the kidney reflexes to the bladder reflexes, revealing the internal flow of urine and the ability to move on.

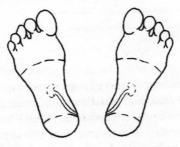

Figure 16.11 The ureter reflexes.

The upper arms

The upper arm reflexes (Figure 16.12) extend along the outer edges of the balls of both feet, from the bases of the little toes to the waistlines of the feet. The lower halves of the upper arms pick up on how communications are being embraced within relationships, while the upper halves reveal the willingness to let go of those who need to be emotionally free, especially within the family. The upper arms help to reach out and welcome new beginnings. These reflexes show the extent to which individuals believe in themselves. They *swell* when wishing to break free from being tied to the family, or develop *hard skin* to show how difficult it is to escape perceived emotional obligations. Massaging these reflexes (p. 276) encourages the release of unnecessary emotional attachments so that everybody can enjoy their own space.

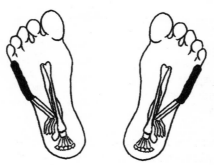

Figure 16.12 The upper arm reflexes.

The lumbar vertebrae

The lumbar vertebrae reflexes (Figure 16.13), extending along the bony arches from the waistline of the feet to the junctions of the insteps and heels, reveal the amount of support and backup within personal relationships to create an awareness of what's going on in the background. These reflexes *bulge* when looking for extra backup and support or *sink* when thinking that nobody cares. Massage these reflexes well to provide the recipient with the courage to back themselves, especially when feeling under attack.

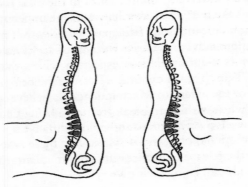

Figure 16.13 The lumbar reflexes.

Insight

'Bad' backs are common in the lower middle back, mirroring 'bad' relationships, or the 'bad' taste left in the mouth, or 'bad' management when wishing to be creative. Any of these can be eased through reflexology.

The digestive process

Reflexology calms down the whole digestive process, making it so much easier to deal with daily events and cope with everything on one's plate. As circumstances become more palatable, the sense of taste improves, while challenging dilemmas become a pleasure to chew over, more satisfying to swallow and more gratifying to deal with. Relationships become noticeably more loving and accepting, making the thrill of being together something to be savoured. Massaging the digestive reflexes takes a huge weight off the mind and body, replacing it with a much healthier intake, a heartier appetite and a rush of renewed energy ensuring that the recipient enjoys their life to the full.

Insight

The journey of food from the mouth to the anus mimics the ability to take in life's experiences, chew them over, stomach them, analyse them, draw from past experiences for greater understanding and then derive the best of each situation, letting go of any wasteful energy.

Think only the best, be only the best,
Do only the best, relate only the best,
Expect only the best.

10 QUESTIONS TO CONSIDER

1 Which thoughts do the fourth toes and lower insteps pick up on?

2 Which parts of the body are they energetically related to?

3 What is the element that is affected by what is going on within relationships?

4 Which colour reveals the amount of joy and happiness being derived from life?

5 Where are the mouth, small intestine, ileo-caecal valve and appendix reflexes? What influences their functioning?

6 Which female reproductive organs are related to the fourth toes and where are their reflexes?

7 What's the role of the kidneys and where do they reflect on the feet?

8 Why are the upper arm reflexes so significant?

9 How are the lumbar vertebrae reflexes connected to the fourth toes?

10 How can reflexology assist digestion?

10 THINGS TO REMEMBER

1   *The fourth toes are the communication and relationship toes.*

2   *These toes resonate to the colour orange and the element of water.*

3   *The mouth, teeth and gums are linked to the fourth toes, revealing the impact of words, whether unspoken or spoken; they also play a role in decision making.*

4   *Massaging the small intestine area reflexes, on the lower halves of the sole insteps, encourages a balanced give and take within relationships.*

5   *Palpating the ileo-caecal valve reflexes, on the outer corner of the right lower sole instep, ensures the onward movement of the more wasteful aspects of life for eventual elimination.*

6   *Stimulating the colon reflexes, bordering the lower halves of the insteps, persuades the mind and body to let go of remnants from the past.*

7   *Evoking the kidney reflexes, immediately beneath the adrenal gland reflexes, initiates the process of letting go of worked-through thoughts and emotions.*

8   *Coaxing the ovary reflexes, on the outer lower corner of both insteps, stimulates creativity and generates new concepts.*

9   *The lower middle back reflexes reveal the amount of backing and support in relationships, as well as what is going on in the background.*

10 *Reflexology calms the whole digestive tract leading to increased energy and greater enjoyment of life.*

The little toes and heels

In this chapter you will learn:
- *about the influence of family and society*
- *why and when to let go*
- *how to make better progress.*

Family and social belief systems

The height and stature of the little toes show the impact that
family and social belief systems have on an individual's standing
in society. When relaxed, they are upright and well-sized, revealing
that the individual feels good about who and what they are and
proud to be unique. They *bow*, from kowtowing to the family,
while keeping the authentic self is kept in the background.

Although small, don't be misled by their appearance. They are
energetically linked to four major systems, namely the excretory,
reproductive, skeletal and muscular, as well as the little fingers,
jaw and pelvis. With such incredible power when 'push comes to
shove', these toes make sure that individuals get on in their own
way, which the heels are quick to pick up on. Together the little
toes and heels disclose innermost feelings about being unique along
with the opportunities to move on and grow and develop into
the most incredible individual. By grounding the body's energies,
they 'keep the feet on the ground', with the solidarity of earth.
Providing a firm foundation for the establishment of roots, with

the freedom to come and go and even change direction whenever necessary. The colour that they resonate to is a deep passionate red, filled to the brim with energy for life to be lived to the full. The little toes, along with the heels, balance the feet and act as shock absorbers. Reflexology puts the 'spring into the step', making ongoing progress possible!

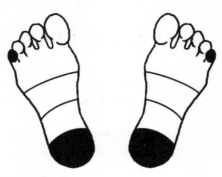

Figure 17.1 The little toes and heels.

The heels

Any self-imposed limitations, especially those induced by the family and society, hold both mind and body back, the effect of which immediately shows up on the heels. They *bruise* when past hurts get in the way; *crack* up when feeling divided or pulled in many directions; *harden* when experiencing difficulty in making progress; become *heavy* when life is heavy-going; their rims *toughen* from constantly dragging or digging in the heels; become *painful* when going through unpleasant growth experiences; get *rough* when the going gets tough; become *spongy* from being a 'softie' and giving in too easily; appear *insignificant* when holding back or having to tread carefully or when 'walking on egg shells'. The colours that show up here draw attention to the emotions that are concerned (Chapter 8). Concentrate on the heels for all *muscular* and *skeletal disorders*, for the inner strength to enjoy the fullness of life; also for *accidents*, to eliminate needless recklessness; for *calluses*, to bring out true authenticity; for *fistulas*, to find a direct outlet for the nonsense that gets in the way; for *plantar warts*, to ease changes in direction; for *rheumatism*, to release past resentment; for *ulcers*, for greater belief in oneself; and for *muscle weakness*, to make it easier to move ahead. Massage the heels well to spur the recipient on with an enthusiasm that defies limitations.

Insight

Do you ever dig in your heels or clench your jaw? It's all linked to the little toes, as well as feelings of security and flexibility within the family and society. To overcome this, become the most exciting and interesting individual that you have the pleasure to know!

The jaw

The *jaw reflexes* (Figure 17.2), situated along the underneath edges of all toe pads, reveal the amount of confidence in being unique. The jaw's solidity provides a firm, yet mobile platform, for ideas to be bounced off, while its flexibility relies on the courage to speak up and be truthful. Intense restraints due to extreme uncertainty and a fear of what others may say and think result in a build-up of tension and tautness that adversely affects its joints. Massage these reflexes (p. 230) for greater flexibility and spend additional time on them for all *jaw disorders*, including *acne*, to neutralize the inner fury and establish the assurance needed to face the world with unique concepts; for *ageing*, to set the mind and body free from worn-out belief systems; for *migraine headaches*, to release the mind from intense pressure; for *paralysis*, to deal with the terror of moving ahead; and for *Parkinson's disease*, to firm up a shaky foundation. Reflexology provides the flexibility and confidence to 'open the mouth' and voice what's on the mind whenever there's an opportunity for self-improvement.

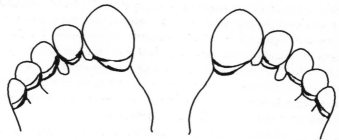

Figure 17.2 The jaw reflexes.

The skin

The sensitivity of the skin reveals everything that is going on 'beneath the surface'. Its colour, especially on the feet, highlights emotions that surface from time to time, according to the type of subconscious mind chatter and, as the mind hops from one theme to another, the colours constantly change (Chapter 8). Reflexology encourages a shift in consciousness and a more tolerant approach to life, clearing the skin of any exasperating memories from the past. When calm, there's less likelihood of a bad reaction to irritating and irrational situations or of letting things get 'under the skin'.

The skeleton

The solid skeleton (Figure 17.3) reveals the substance within, providing the means to be incredibly resourceful and strong enough to deal with the 'ups and downs' of life. The skeletal reflexes, being so extensively mapped out throughout both feet, supply invaluable clues as to inner security and outer mobility. The stronger the bones, the greater the confidence and vice versa, so feeling proud of being 'one of a kind' strengthens the bones, whereas concern about being inadequate, without a 'leg to stand on', weakens the bones, subsequently denying the body of its strength and resourcefulness; this makes it really difficult to keep going, especially if there's a 'bone of contention' or a tendency to 'pick at one another's bones'. *Breaking* a bone often confirms the need to break away from somebody or something, the location revealing who or what it is. Massaging the feet eases *bursitis*, by facilitating any change in direction, no matter how arduous or infuriating the circumstances; as well as *osteoporosis*, replacing the 'oh poor us' mentality and tendency to rely on others with enhanced inner substance. Bones that protrude on the feet exhibit a need for more space or additional support and backup; note where these protrusions are to get the gist of what's going on. Reflexology is an excellent way of bolstering inner strength and of replenishing personal resourcefulness, especially when the present one isn't going the way it should or anywhere in particular. It helps in making the most of any adversity, using the perceived misfortune as a guideline to sketch out another plan.

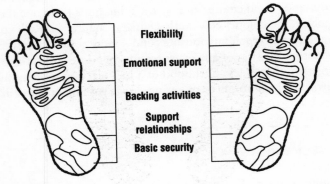

Flexibility

Emotional support

Backing activities

Support relationships

Basic security

Figure 17.3 The skeletal reflexes.

The muscles

It's thanks to the flexibility and adaptability of the *muscles* (Figure 17.4) that the body can expand every time an innovative concept is implemented; this, in turn, helps personal growth and development, physically, mentally, emotionally and spiritually. Being more open-minded relaxes the muscles and encourages them to be more flexible, whereas very set beliefs and extreme fear make them taut, rigid and often unforgiving. Reflexology entices the recipient to extend themselves beyond self-imposed limitations, so that the muscles have the opportunity to stretch with ease. This allows way-out and extraordinary thoughts to be implemented without fear of the consequences. Massaging the feet reminds the muscles of their inborn strength, tone, power, as well as the impetus required for the next step towards self-empowerment. Muscles love being soothed and respond exceptionally well to reflexology.

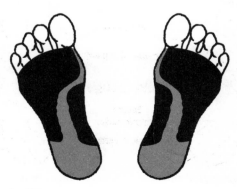

Figure 17.4 The muscular reflexes.

The pelvic bone

The pelvic bone reflexes (Figure 17.5) occupy the bulk of the heel
pads, top and bottom. The solidarity of the pelvic area allows the
mind and body to pivot when changing direction, so that they can
energetically stride out for greater personal progress and enhanced
wellbeing.

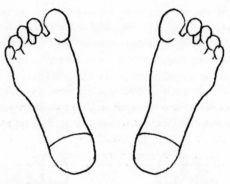

Figure 17.5 The pelvic bone reflexes.

> The joy of the spirit indicates its strength.

The hips

The body is propelled through life by the hips, which provide
the motivation and incentive to move ahead and get going.

The prominence of these reflexes is obvious, since they are the outer ankle bones (Figure 17.6). The small firm swellings, just beneath them, reflect the ball and socket joints at the tops of the legs. Together they reveal the ability to move forwards, backwards or sideways. They *swell* when begrudgingly overburdened or weighed down and develop *broken blood vessels* when unhappy at the lack of progress. Massaging these reflexes eases changes in direction through greater understanding of what it is that the soul requires.

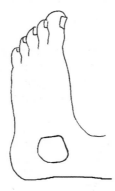

Figure 17.6 The hip reflexes.

Insight

The pelvis provides a secure base from which to move, while the hips provide the thrust to get going. Massaging the heels and outer ankle bones, therefore, can provide the flexibility to change direction whenever required.

The buttocks

The buttocks are the seat of power and their reflexes (Figure 17.7), on the rounded aspect of the heels, beneath the outer ankle bones, reflect the amount of influence an individual has over the direction of their life. *Flabby* buttocks imply a lack of control, usually from being so reliant on others for basic security, while exceptionally *taut* buttocks suggest that an extremely tight rein and firm control is being kept, particularly on the 'purse strings'. Massaging the buttock reflexes (p. 280) empowers the authentic self so that it can come to the forefront and be noticed.

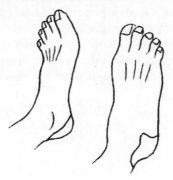

Figure 17.7 The buttock reflexes.

Insight

Tone up the 'glutes'! It's an excellent way to boost the seat of power! However, avoid overdoing it because really tight 'butts' reflect too tight a control on life.

The rectum

The arc-shaped rectum reflexes (Figure 17.8), on the inner surfaces of both heels, represent the competence to finally let go of anything that's a waste of time and energy. They also reveal the willingness to release the rougher aspects of life, so that these are no longer entertained in the mind or body. The rectum reflexes may *swell* from being constipated or when fearful of letting go; they *sink*, when on the run, generally to escape current circumstances usually through *diarrhoea*; they turn *red*, possibly from *haemorrhoids* that arise from a fear of deadlines; or *distend* with *red* tinges, when there's a likelihood of *diverticulitis*. Milking these reflexes helps to alleviate any discontent at being unnecessarily encumbered, strained or suppressed, while reflexology provides the necessary ongoing relief from having to carry such a load of nonsense.

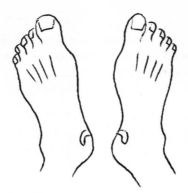

Figure 17.8 The rectum reflexes.

The anus

The reflexes for the anus (Figure 17.9) are small palpable indentations, midway between the inner ankle bones and tips of the inside heels. Soothing these reflexes does away with the need to be so crude when feeling exceptionally frustrated about hanging on to issues for an unacceptable length of time.

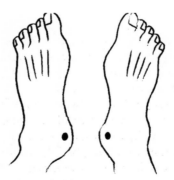

Figure 17.9 The anus reflexes.

The bladder

The bladder reflexes (Figure 17.10), the fleshy mounds on the inside edges of the insteps, at the junction with the heels, reflect the bladder's ability to act as a reservoir for worked-through thoughts and emotions, until they can be conveniently released. They tend to *swell* quite considerably when unhappy about an intimate relationship or partner, hence feeling 'pissed or pee-ed off'. Gently caress these fleshy mounds (p. 286) to create greater comfort and to be more accommodating with their situation or partner's downfalls. Additional attention is required for all *bladder disorders*, to expel old concerns that play havoc with the mind and emotions. Reflexology relaxes the bladder so that every last drop can be released when the time comes.

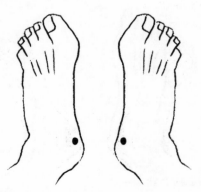

Figure 17.10 The bladder reflexes.

The urethra

The *urethra* reflexes extend from the fleshy mounds on the inner aspects of the feet to the slight indentations, midway between the inside ankle bones and tips of the heels on females (Figure 17.11), and to the tips of the heels on males (Figure 17.12). The urethra consists of two muscular sphincters, which control the final release of old energy that has been well processed. This ability is temporarily lost when under extreme pressure or in a life-threatening situation over which there seems to be no control. This can lead to *incontinence* in the elderly or *bed wetting* in youngsters, the latter being linked to tension at home due to the father's circumstances. Massaging these reflexes re-establishes control of the comings and goings of the mind, making it physically viable to go with the flow.

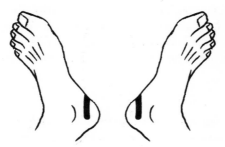

Figure 17.11 The female urethra reflexes.

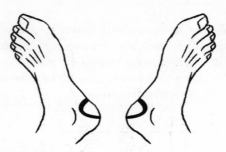

Figure 17.12 *The male urethra reflexes.*

The lower reproductive parts

The reflexes for the lower reproductive organs and glands (Figure 17.13) are reflected onto the inner triangular areas of the heels, representing both masculine and feminine traits, which everybody has. The male energy comes from the father's sperm and the female energy from the mother's egg, which is why the reproductive organs represent everything to do with being either male or female. The reflexes appear *bruised* when hurt from being taken advantage of, or from not receiving recognition because of being a specific gender, while small *broken blood vessels* indicate extreme unhappiness at being perceivably abused, be it mentally, emotionally, physically or spiritually. Reflexology brings about the realization that there are no 'opposites', only 'oppo-sames', with each gender being reliant on the other for the balance in life. One without the other would bring life to a standstill.

> **Insight**
> Everybody has both male and female energies that stem from the sperm of the father and the ovum of the mother. It's acknowledging the roles of both parents and their roles, regardless of the circumstances, that keeps these energies well balanced.

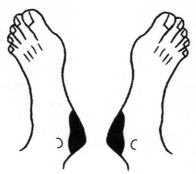

Figure 17.13 The reproductive reflexes.

The uterus

The uterus, better known as the 'womb', reflects the home, since it's the first place of residence from conception to birth. Its reflexes (Figure 17.14), on the lower inside edges of both sole and side insteps, reflect the female principle, revealing all that is 'going on' or not 'going on' at home. They *swell* when pregnant with new concepts or with a baby; turn *red* when disappointed or frustrated at the lack of acceptance or recognition of creative

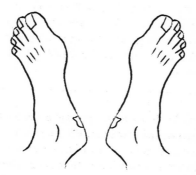

Figure 17.14 The uterus reflexes.

notions; look *battered* when unable to get ahead because of social beliefs, or develop a *cut*, when there's been a severance of home ties or possibly a *hysterectomy*, should this be an issue. Pay additional attention to these reflexes for any *menstrual, infertility* or *pregnancy disorder*, to resolve outstanding issues with certain women and to create greater affiliation with being female. Reflexology brings peace into the home, making everybody feel well loved and lovingly nurtured.

The vagina

The vagina reflexes (Figure 17.15), on the hollows between the inner ankle bones and heel tips, reveal the reaction at having to meet social obligations, along with all that comes with being a female. *Broken blood vessels* or *bruising* over these reflexes can be indicative of sexual abuse, be it physical, mental or emotional. Massaging these reflexes (p. 283) creates pride about being a woman.

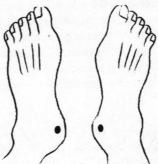

Figure 17.15 The vagina reflexes.

The male reproductive organs

The male reproductive organs and glands, situated on the inside heels of both feet (Figure 17.16), reflect the man's perception of himself and his designated role in life. They also reveal how well he functions as a man, whether a gentle man or not, and how well he performs sexually. Spend extra time on these reflexes for male issues, such as *impotence*, so that he feels 'important' and can 'rise' to the occasion as and when required. Reflexology helps men to realize that they don't have to be a menace to get their point across and that it's okay to just be their charming selves!

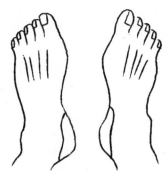

Figure 17.16 The male reproductive reflexes.

The testes

The position of the testes reflexes (Figure 17.17), on or near the tips of the inside parts of the heels varies because of the testes' tendency to hang lower down when it's hot so that they can stay cool, while a hasty retreat is made back into the body, as soon as it gets too cold. The testes continually 'test their way' through life; their sperm count is symbolic of their perceived ability to make a worthwhile contribution to society's progress. Stimulating these reflexes helps them get on and do what they need to do, so that they feel good about being the man they are.

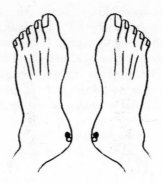

Figure 17.17 The testes reflexes.

The base of the back

The solid reflexes of the lower back (Figure 17.18), on the bony insteps that curve in and under the inner ankle bones, reflect the amount of basic backing and support available when expanding horizons and exploring new territories. These reflexes *distend* when reaching out for more support, especially financial backing, and *sink* when there's insufficient money or a drain on personal resources. Bolster these reflexes (p. 243) to reinforce the recipient's belief in their own worth, as well as for *lower back pain*, to relieve the hurt at not having the backup necessary to get on with what the soul requires. Reflexology enriches mind, body and soul to such an extent that all the resources become available, through faith and by asking the universe for assistance and support. This comes from having made a worthwhile contribution to the betterment of others.

Insight
The lower back and little toes are energetically connected. They can both be an absolute pain when no progress is being made or when there are insufficient funds. This pain can spread to the feet and may even cause numbness during exceptionally difficult times.

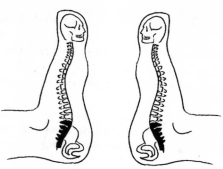

Figure 17.18 The lower back reflexes.

Life can be understood backwards, but must be lived forwards!

10 QUESTIONS TO CONSIDER

1   What do the height and stature of the little toes signify?

2   Which major systems of the body are connected to the little toes?

3   Which element and colour influence them the most? How do these reveal what is going on in the family and society?

4   Where are the jaw reflexes?

5   Describe your heels. What do you like and dislike about them? Is there anything you can do to change or improve them?

6   What does the strength of the bones signify? What impact do the muscles have on the body and feet?

7   Where are the pelvic bone, hip, buttocks, rectum and anus reflexes situated?

8   What should the bladder reflexes look like?

9   Which lower reproductive organ and gland reflexes are situated on the inside of both ankles?

10 What causes changes in the lower back reflexes and why?

10 THINGS TO REMEMBER

1   *The little 'family and society' toes represent thoughts about personal security, an individual's perceived role and status within the family and society, the impression of which is reflected onto the heels.*

2   *The little toes and heels resonate with the colour red and the element of earth.*

3   *The jaw reflexes, on the lower edges of each toe pad, reveal the belief in personal concepts and the courage to speak one's mind.*

4   *Massaging the heels stimulates the skeletal system, enhancing inner strength, along with the ability to 'stand on one's own two feet'.*

5   *Palpating the heels stimulates the muscular system, augmenting flexibility for the expansive implementation of ideas, to ensure the ongoing movement of life.*

6   *The pelvic bone occupies most of the heel pads, providing a solid foundation to move forward, as well as a pivot for a complete change in direction.*

7   *Palpating the inner heels either calms and balances or stimulates and activates the rectum, anus, urethra and bladder.*

8   *Rubbing the outer heels fortifies the hips, for a secure foundation to keep going, while tightening or loosening the buttocks to adjust the amount of control required to make progress.*

9   *Both male and female reproductive systems are reflected onto the inner triangular areas of both heels; when massaged they balance, stimulate or calm the sexual energies.*

10 *The lower back is reflected onto the bony ridges underneath both inner ankles, reflecting the support and backing available to move forward into new experiences.*

Pregnancy

In this chapter you will learn:
- *about reflexology's role in pregnancy*
- *about the benefits to all concerned*
- *how to detect a baby's presence.*

Before conception

Before falling pregnant, both parents should ideally receive reflexology on a regular basis, for at least a year. For the father-to-be it helps to ensure stronger, healthier sperm and prepares him physically, mentally, emotionally and spiritually, giving him the inner strength and confidence to support the mother-to-be throughout the pregnancy. For the mother-to-be it creates a much more conducive womb environment, boosts her resourcefulness, gives her greater awareness of her role as a mother and increases her intuitive abilities, all of which make the unborn baby feel most welcome. With her womb being so receptive and providing such a loving space, the unborn baby is able to grow and develop to its full potential.

Insight

Reflexology is enormously beneficial to both mother and unborn baby. They both thrive on the calming and harmonizing effects of the mother's feet being massaged, especially when it's loving and gentle.

During pregnancy

During pregnancy the reproductive reflexes enlarge or form a shadow in the shape of the developing embryo (Figure 18.1) around six weeks after conception. This embryonic shape is generally seen on one of the uterine reflexes on the inside edge of one foot. In 80 per cent of pregnancies, if the swelling is on the right instep, the baby is a boy, and, if it's on the left foot, it's more likely to be a girl; should it be on both then there's a possibility of twins, although this is by no means an accurate prediction.

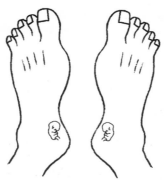

Figure 18.1 Around six weeks of pregnancy.

Insight

The ability to conceive has its roots way back in time, so it helps to know what one's ancestors went through. Understanding their situations makes it easier to unravel the mystery as why some couples conceive when not wishing to, while others struggle for years. Either way, it's great for couples to massage each other's feet.

Both the mother-to-be and her unborn baby thrive on reflexology, while the father-to-be becomes more supportive and understanding, making him feel more competent. When massaging the feet of a pregnant woman, the touch should be particularly gentle, light and loving, especially over her womb reflexes. The other areas that require additional attention are the breast, pelvis and vagina reflexes so that they can undergo their changes naturally. If the father-to-be regularly massages his partner's feet, he can get more involved by doing something really worthwhile. It not only establishes a much healthier relationship between the parents-to-be, but also creates a closer bond with the unborn baby. Reflexology during pregnancy helps in dealing with *morning sickness*, by reassuring the mother-to-be that she can and will cope; eases *back pain*, providing greater inner strength and support; prevents or soothes *varicose veins*, by ensuring that the pregnancy is pleasurable; and enhances the *blood flow*, particularly to the womb; this ensures a good supply of vital life force energies for the healthy development of the baby. It keeps the close-knit family unit well, content and happy.

As the baby starts to show on the body, its outline becomes increasingly visible on the corresponding areas of the feet. At times, these reflexes can be so clear that the baby's body parts can be identified, particularly the head and buttocks (Figure 18.2). Should the baby be in a breech or unnatural position, try rotating the mother-to-be's little toes, since this has been known to encourage the unborn baby to turn. Reflexology makes sure that both the mother-to-be and unborn baby are well cared for, so that, when the time comes, they feel completely at home with one another.

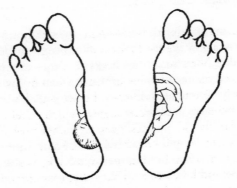

Figure 18.2 The reflection of the developing foetus.

Insight

Regular reflexology throughout pregnancy relaxes the mother-to-be's mind and body; it consequently facilitates and eases the birth process. After the birth the mother is more likely to feel great! Remember to caress the baby's feet too.

During childbirth

As soon as the baby's head engages in the pelvic cavity, small rounded swellings are often visible on the edges of the heels of both feet, near the insteps (Figure 18.3).

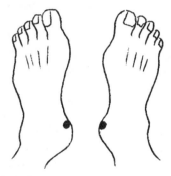

Figure 18.3 Engaged head of the developing foetus.

Reflexology during childbirth is excellent, especially when it's the father-to-be massaging the feet! Not only is it calming, relaxing and reassuring for both but it also keeps the expectant father well occupied and makes him feel useful, instead of just standing around helplessly. With the mother-to-be being able to relax, she can breathe more easily and more deeply, which is helpful when giving birth naturally. Sometimes, even when her cervix is fully dilated, she may not be quite ready to push. She is more likely to be ready to push, when her big toes pull back, as she puts her own thoughts behind her, while all her other toes extend forwards, as she puts all her energy into giving birth to the baby. All in all, reflexology makes the whole experience of childbirth the enjoyable and natural experience that it should be.

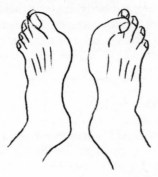

Figure 18.4 The mother-to-be ready to actively participate in the childbirth process.

> **Insight**
> The word 'labour' instils an image of long drawn out, hard work. The miracle of childbirth doesn't have to be like this! Encourage expectant mothers not to listen to these horror stories and remain relaxed and focused on everything positive.

After childbirth

When both parents continue to receive reflexology after the birth of their baby, they are far more relaxed and stay much calmer, which is exceptionally reassuring for the baby. With no distress signals coming from either parent, the baby has no reason to cry. Babies love having their feet massaged, especially while being fed; their tiny feet are well positioned for this, being so affectionately cradled in their mother's arms. Reflexology helps the whole family adapt to their exciting new circumstances, ensuring a loving home environment, filled with complete appreciation for one another.

10 QUESTIONS TO CONSIDER

1   How can reflexology assist the parents-to-be before falling pregnant?

2   What are the benefits of feet being regularly massaged during pregnancy?

3   How does the baby benefit?

4   What can reflexology do for the prospective father?

5   Where on the feet can the embryo reflexes be seen around six to eight weeks after conception?

6   How can reflexology assist with a breach pregnancy?

7   Why is it a good idea for the father-to-be to massage his partner's feet during childbirth?

8   What happens to the toes when the mother-to-be is ready to give birth?

9   Why is it so beneficial for all family members to have their feet massaged after the baby is born?

10 How confident are you about giving a pregnant lady reflexology now that you've read this information?

10 THINGS TO REMEMBER

1   *Regular reflexology can enhance the chances of conception.*

2   *Massaging the feet before falling pregnant makes the mother-to-be's body more receptive and a welcoming environment for the incoming baby.*

3   *Before conception, reflexology assists the father-to-be in producing stronger sperm and prepares him for his future role.*

4   *During pregnancy the shape of the early embryo is often seen on the uterus reflex on the inside heels of one or both feet.*

5   *Use a very light touch over the extra-sensitive areas of the uterus, breasts, pelvis and vagina reflexes when giving reflexology to a pregnant woman.*

6   *Reflexology enhances the blood flow to the womb, ensuring a continual flow of life force energies to the baby.*

7   *If the baby is in the breech position, rotating the mother's little toes may encourage it to turn.*

8   *Giving reflexology during childbirth calms, reassures and relaxes the mother-to-be, making the birth process so much easier.*

9   *When the mother-to-be is ready to push, her big toes pull back as she puts her own thoughts behind her, while all her other toes extend forwards, as she channels her energy into giving birth to the baby.*

10   *After the birth, reflexology can help both parents remain relaxed and calm.*

19

The technique

In this chapter you will learn:
* *four simple movements*
* *how much pressure to use*
* *the effects of each technique.*

Four simple movements

There are four simple movements, each of which can be adjusted to meet the ever-changing needs of the recipient. This means that every treatment can be personalized to suit every individual's needs. The four techniques are the **rotation technique**, which creates an energetic link with the universe; the **caterpillar movement,** which improves the physique by enhancing inner strength; the **stroking or milking method** that soothes emotions so that the individual can feel better about themselves and others; and the **feather or healing caress**, which reacquaints the recipient with their authentic self. Knowing exactly how much pressure to apply is an intuitive process that cannot be taught; you will just know when to be firm, or when to pull back until there's little or no physical contact. To get a feel for these movements, try practising them on your hand first to gain the confidence to do it on others.

Insight
Hands move instinctively when massaging the feet, unless the mind gets in the way! Trusting the intuition is the ideal way to get the best and most beneficial reactions.

Technique 1 – rotation

Gently rest the tip of any digit onto the reflex (Figure 19.1) and
apply slight pressure; hold for a while, then very slowly release.
A delightful tingling sensation may be felt as energy floods back
into this area. Without moving your digit, gently gyrate it and keep
doing this for as long as necessary. Now allow your digit to rest
very lightly on the skin's surface for a short while before moving it
on to the next reflex. This rotation technique is ideal for opening
up and activating all energy channels, soothing fraught nerves and
creating greater awareness of oneself and others while, at the same
time, balancing and harmonizing the whole being.

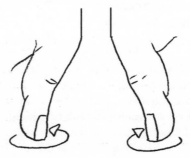

Figure 19.1 The rotation technique.

Technique 2 – caterpillar movement

Place the tip of your thumb gently onto the reflex and then
slowly lower your thumb onto its pad (Figure 19.2) 'jerking
it' fractionally forward; now raise your thumb up onto its tip
again before 'dropping' it back down onto its pad. Keep rocking
your thumb, up and down, as you gradually move it, bit by bit,
either backwards, to unravel the past, or forwards, to ensure

that progress is made. 'Walking' the thumbs, in this way, eases muscular tension, relieves physical distress and alleviates aches and pains, while, at the same time, encouraging an improved approach to life.

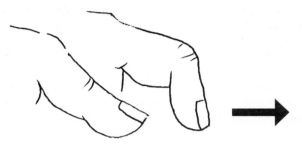

Figure 19.2 The caterpillar movement.

Insight

It's impossible to wash, touch or apply pressure to any part of the body or feet without evoking a reaction. So it is that when the feet are touched during reflexology, the pressure applied should vary to suit individual physical, emotional and spiritual needs.

Technique 3 – stroking or milking

This technique usually follows the rotation and caterpillar movements. Stroke or milk the reflex, by placing both thumbs on the skin's surface. While applying slight pressure, make long, reassuring and soothing sweeps (Figure 19.3), thumb over thumb, on top of the reflexes, as though gently squeezing a tube of toothpaste. This stroking or milking method soothes disturbed emotions, eliminates disruptive feelings, boosts self-confidence and creates inner harmony.

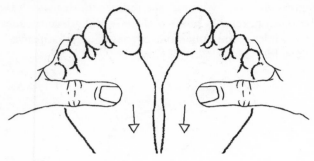

Figure 19.3 The stroking or milking method 1.

Alternatively do this technique with shorter caressing movements (Figure 19.4).

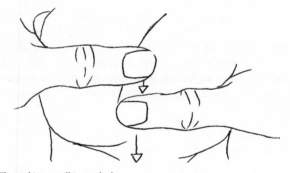

Figure 19.4 The stroking or milking method 2.

Technique 4 – feathering or healing caress

This is the final movement of each sequence. Very lightly stroke the skin's surface, by alternating your digits (Figure 19.5), either in generous scoops or minuscule strokes, as though you are caressing the energies just above the skin's surface. These movements reconnect the spirit with its purpose and bring the recipient's true essence to the fore, helping them to get to know themselves and others better.

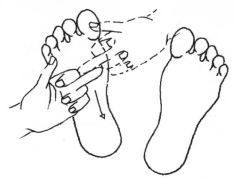

Figure 19.5 The feathering or healing caress.

Insight

Experiment on one of your hands, using different fingers and applying various pressures, to get a feel for the wide range of sensations that can be experienced through touch.

The soul came to earth for the richest experience, not the poorest, for the most, not the least.

10 QUESTIONS TO CONSIDER

1 *How many basic movements are they in reflexology?*

2 *Name each technique and describe what it does for mind, body and soul.*

3 *Why should the approach vary when massaging the feet?*

4 *How much pressure should be applied?*

5 *What is the best way to practise the technique?*

6 *How are the energy channels of the mind, body and soul opened and activated?*

7 *How can tension, pain and distress be eased by reflexology?*

8 *Which is the most soothing technique?*

9 *In reflexology, how is the soul reconnected with its true spirit?*

10 *Why is it important for you to get to know yourself better?*

10 THINGS TO REMEMBER

1   Since every treatment and recipient is unique, your touch and technique should vary according to what's required.

2   There are four main types of touch techniques: rotation, caterpillar movement, milking and feathering.

3   For the rotation touch, apply light pressure to the reflex using any digit and gently circle it over the point of contact, then let it rest lightly for a while, without moving.

4   The rotation movement is ideal for opening up and activating a reflex and creating a link with the universe.

5   For the caterpillar movement, the thumbs are used to 'walk' over the reflex.

6   The caterpillar movement eases tension, aches and pains and encourages greater inner strength, enhancing the physical aspect of the healing.

7   For the milking touch use longer sweeps, thumb over thumb, applying slight pressure.

8   The milking touch is used after the caterpillar movement to soothe disturbed emotions and encourage a release of whatever is no longer required.

9   The feathering touch involves very light stroking, accentuating the spiritual aspect of healing.

10 Use the feathering touch with alternating digits after the caterpillar and milking, to reconnect with the essence of the spirit within.

20

What to expect

In this chapter you will learn:
- *about the sensations felt*
- *about less common reactions*
- *about pleasurable after-effects.*

The sensations experienced

As the recipient drifts into the exquisite alpha level of consciousness, they remain acutely aware of everything that is going on around them, but are so pleasantly detached that they couldn't care less! In this way, they never need to lose control, despite appearing to be in a deep sleep. With their mind and body so still, they can fully appreciate the fantastic sensations felt during the reflexology massage. Everybody's experience is totally different, so it's impossible to predict how the recipient is going to react; but if they are aware of what could happen, their mind is put to rest. This means that they willingly let go and, therefore, can benefit more fully from all that reflexology has to offer.

Some common responses are *heat loss*, as the body relaxes and 'let's off steam'; *extreme tenderness*, despite the light touch, as hurt feelings surface; a *sinking feeling*, as mind and body drop off into a space of peace; a *floating sensation*, as burdens dissipate and a weight is taken off their whole being; *twitching* and *jerking* as a sudden surge of energy reaches previously deprived, tense areas; *pins and needles* or *numbness* in the hands coming from letting go of the difficulty in handling certain circumstances; *snoring* as deeply suppressed emotions finally escape; *visions of colours*, ranging from subdued, subtle hues to gorgeous bright tints, even though the eyes are closed.

Insight

There are no right or wrong reactions to reflexology. Whatever is experienced is exactly what is required at the time. This is also why two treatments are never the same!

Less common reactions

Less common reactions include *plucking hand movements*, when uncertain about how to handle current circumstances; *out-of-body experiences*, as the soul temporarily leaves the body for a different viewpoint; *recall* of previous life situations; *singing* out loud. Some may even get the feeling that a murky lining of emotional trash is being pulled from their insides, like a piece of material. Just remember that whatever happens, it is absolutely ideal for the person concerned, no matter how peculiar or unexpected it may be.

While the feet are being massaged, the breathing can become so shallow that, at times, it is almost indiscernible, but don't panic! The recipient drifts into other spheres of consciousness, which is why it is necessary to ask them to take three deep breaths, at the end of the session, to bring them back. They are often reluctant to leave this space of pure bliss, so give them a little time. Better still, if they have had their feet massaged in their own bed, then all they need to do is roll over and drift back into this amazing state of consciousness, emerging in their own time, feeling great.

Healing occurs when going from a state of discomfort and distress, to one of harmony and ease.

Pleasurable after-effects

Always explain to the recipient that any reaction to reflexology is a good reaction, since it works with, and not against, the manifestations of illness. The cycles of 'dis-ease' need to be completed before healing can begin, which is why the recipient may feel worse, rather than better, after having their feet massaged. Reflexology should not, therefore, be a one-off treatment, but rather received on a regular basis of at least once a week.

Fortunately most people feel absolutely fantastic after a session; full of energy along with a huge sense of relief! It means that a favourable energy shift has taken place in their body, with a corresponding and much-needed change of mind. The renewed enthusiasm for life makes it easier to think more clearly, with the recipient becoming far more tolerant and much more reasonable; they also sleep so much better and wake up feeling refreshed. If they remember their dreams, some incredible insight can be gained, along with some additional spiritual guidance. Being more conscious of their mind, body and spirit, means that they can tune in and care more for their wellbeing and, in the process, attain a deeper understanding of their soul's purpose. A much-improved quality of life can then be enjoyed!

> **Insight**
> Even after the treatment has come to an end, the body continues to balance and heal itself. Allowing the body to respond naturally and in its own way accelerates the healing process.

Excellent signs of healing

Massaging the feet effectively evacuates mind and body of old, outdated beliefs and detrimental habits, making the way clear for a fresh start and a much more meaningful approach to life. Although the effects of this cleansing process could initially be disturbing, exhausting or disruptive, once over, there is a fantastic feeling of liberation and release.

Any of the following are excellent signs that the body is helping itself to better health: *headaches*, as everything 'comes to a head' and solutions are found; *high temperatures*, when 'letting off steam' and giving vent to heated emotions; *increased perspiration*, as old fears, anxiety and concern are flushed out; *runny eyes*, as unshed tears are unleashed and any sadness in sight is washed away; *cold* or *runny nose*, as past irritations are evacuated; *skin rashes* or *eruptions*, as irrational, boiling emotions that 'got under the skin' come to the surface to escape; a more *virulent vaginal discharge* in women, as exasperating female issues are dispensed with; *increased urination*, as the body is relieved of worked-through thoughts and emotions; *frequent, easier defecation* as the wasteful remnants of life's processes are eliminated; temporary *diarrhoea*, as unnecessary nonsense and unreasonable pressure are removed; *vivid recall of dreams*, for a greater understanding of what's going on. This flushing-through process is accelerated when plenty of purified water is taken in after the reflexology massage, which also hastens the healing.

Insight

Reflexology can trigger profound emotions, as well as extreme anxiety or even panic attacks, during a treatment. Should this happen, just relax and gently place your thumbs on the solar plexus reflexes, whilst encouraging the recipient to take in long, slow, deep breaths. They'll feel amazing afterwards!

Unusual reactions

Natural stimulants evoke natural responses, so it is impossible to cause any harm with the light, but firm, movements used in reflexology. However, individuals do like to challenge themselves, from time to time, as a test of their own inner strength and resourcefulness, which they do by forcing themselves to deal with the most unexpected, and often perceivably adverse, situations. It's all part of the growth experience. Should horrendous memories come to the fore while the feet are being massaged, the recipient may have what seems like a really alarming reaction. These seemingly 'bad' reactions come from the subconscious arousal of heart-wrenching emotions that can cause *palpitations*, *hyperventilation* or *panic*, indicating a desperate need to release a truly horrific memory.

If this happens, just remain calm and immediately place your thumbs or middle fingers onto the solar plexus reflexes (p. 245), allowing yourself to be intuitively guided into knowing what to do next. Keep telling yourself that every reaction is a good reaction and that, since reflexology is a non-invasive, natural therapy, only dormant issues that were already resident in the body can be brought to the fore. It shouldn't take long for the recipient to calm down, but if it does take a while, be patient and just keep breathing steadily; then once the recipient is more tranquil, continue with the massage. Encourage the recipient to drink more purified water than usual, to flush out all the additional toxins. Also suggest a further treatment, within the next day or two, to balance mind, body and soul. Although this is not a common occurrence, it is best to be aware of what to do, should there ever be an unusual and intense reaction.

Everybody is completely responsible for their own thoughts, actions and reactions.

10 QUESTIONS TO CONSIDER

1 Why is everybody's experience of reflexology so different?

2 Is it possible to predict how a recipient is going to react to treatment?

3 What are some of the more common responses to reflexology?

4 Describe some of the less likely reactions.

5 Why is it important to explain possible side-effects to the recipient?

6 How do most people feel after a reflexology session?

7 How does the body cleanse itself of toxic thoughts and noxious emotions?

8 What helps the recipient flush away the past after a treatment?

9 If there is an unusual or frightening reaction, what can you do?

10 When is it best to massage the feet again after an excessive reaction to reflexology?

10 THINGS TO REMEMBER

1 *Everybody reacts differently to reflexology and there is no right or wrong experience.*

2 *As the recipient drifts off into the alpha state of consciousness, they will remain aware of what is going on around them, but being so deeply relaxed, feel totally detached from it.*

3 *Common responses include a drop in body temperature, sensitivity on certain areas, floating sensations, body twitching and jerking, pins and needles and snoring.*

4 *Less common responses are out-of-body experiences, past life recollections and levitation.*

5 *At the end of each treatment, invite the recipient to take three deep breaths to bring them back to reality.*

6 *The effects of the reflexology can linger long after the treatment finishes.*

7 *Advise the recipient that they may initially feel worse before feeling better.*

8 *An indication that healing is taking place are headaches, heightened emotions, raised temperature, flu-like symptoms, increased urination and defecation, which are all good signs.*

9 *During an unusually strong emotional release, remain calm and gently rest your thumbs or middle fingers on the solar plexus reflexes to reassure the recipient.*

10 *Always encourage the drinking of plenty of purified water after reflexology to help flush out any emotional or physical waste products from the body and facilitate healing.*

21

Preparing for the reflexology massage

In this chapter you will learn:
- *how to make the recipient comfortable*
- *what to tell them*
- *some handy tips.*

Reflexology is a natural healing therapy that is incredibly easy to learn and apply. In fact you already know how to do it because it's an inborn skill that, once rediscovered, can be put to very good use. It's possible that you already massage, rub or stroke your body to ease various forms of discomfort. *Rubbing* the skin soothes bumps, aching joints and weary muscles, or it stimulates dull, numb areas, or is a way of getting the blood moving and warming up the body. *Smearing saliva* over insect bites takes away the itch, or stems minor blood flows over cuts. Then *scratching* is great for relieving irritation, although, at times, it can exacerbate it! Finally it's a natural reaction to *stroke*, *pat* or *hug* others, especially when they are upset or grieving.

So it is with reflexology; you will instinctively know exactly what to do, be it stroking, rubbing, tapping and so on! Just go with the flow! You can't go wrong, particularly when your intent is good and you come from a place of love. Remember, that whatever you are feeling can have a profound impact on the outcome. Reflexology, fortunately, puts things into perspective, making the difference between having a life and living life to the full. So are you ready to begin? Let's get started!

> **Insight**
>
> Don't worry about whether you are going to remember the sequence of what to do and how to do it. Allow your intuition to guide you! To do this it's essential get out of your head and into your heart – it completely changes the energy of the treatment.

Only by venturing into the unknown do you know what you are capable of.

Preparation

Fortunately, you have all that's needed when it comes to doing reflexology; your hands and your heart are the two most essential requirements. Certain standard household goodies can be used to create a more peaceful and relaxed ambiance; these are best prepared in advance, to ensure a warm welcome. Amongst these are a bed, settee, reclining chair or massage couch with several comfortable pillows and fresh, clean coverings; a stool or chair for you to sit on; soft music playing gently in the background; beautiful aromas filling the air; flowers or a plant to bring natural energy into the space; a plastic bowl or foot bath, with warm or hot water to soak the feet, plus some recently laundered towels to dry them with afterwards; some powder, aromatic oils or creams to use during and at the end of the massage; and, finally, two glasses filled with drinking water.

A peaceful setting, in a subdued environment, allows the recipient to escape the frenetic hustle and bustle of the outside world and totally relax. Once they visually let go, by shutting their eyes, however, all external impressions dim into oblivion, making it easier for reflexology to step in and induce inner harmony.

A dimmer switch and/or softly flickering candle light makes everything *visually* so much more pleasing, while whiffs of aromas from an aromatherapy lamp or incense appease the sense of *smell* (see Appendix I), as soothing music creates a *sound* atmosphere (see Appendix III). Place a 'Do not disturb' notice on the door and activate a telephone answering machine or service to prevent any interruptions and avoid losing touch with the recipient. Be conscious of the furnishings in the room, since pastel colours are subconsciously soothing, while exceptionally bright colours either stimulate or can even heighten volatile feelings.

Deep healing requires a willingness and commitment to go deep within.

Communication

When the recipient knows very little or nothing about reflexology, or has never had a session, a simple and clear explanation will help to reassure and relax them. Knowing that it's a trustworthy and natural process helps them to let go, without the fear of being hurt. Also a short explanation of what reflexology is, how it works, what to expect during and after the massage, why they may react the way that they do and why it is advisable for them to drink plenty of water after the massage, means that they then know more or less what to expect.

Those on prescribed medication should advise their specialist of their intention to have reflexology. Appropriate adjustments to the dosage can then be made to cater for any immediate improvements that occur once the healing process has been activated. For the best results, the reflexology session should ideally be just over an hour before any medication is due since this is when the drugs are least effective, making the body more vulnerable and, therefore, more receptive to the natural healing energies. The explanation can be given while the recipient is soaking their feet in the foot spa or plastic bowl.

Comfort

When soaking the recipient's feet in the foot bath, make sure that
the water is pleasantly warm in winter and refreshingly cool in
summer. Consider adding a sprig of lavender or a drop of its oil
to relax the recipient and, when it's particularly warm, a droplet
of peppermint oil, which has a deliciously cooling effect. This is
an ideal time to chat and discover more about the recipient and
for them to gain confidence in you. Hand them a fresh towel to
dry their feet, or do this for them, then invite them to lie as flat
as possible on the bed or couch.

Make them comfortable, by placing one pillow beneath their head
and another one or two pillows under their knees and lower legs,
so that their spine is straight and flat. Place a light sheet over them,
when it's hot, and a warm blanket or, better still, a cosy duvet
when it's cold, since body heat is generally lost as they sink deeper
and deeper into a state of complete relaxation. For ladies wearing
skirts or dresses, for modesty reasons, tuck the blanket between
their knees because their legs do need to be slightly apart to gain
sufficient access to all the reflexes on the feet.

Start by shaking powder into your hand, rub your palms together
and then spread it gently over both feet, going in between their toes.

This not only facilitates the massage but also helps the recipient feel less self-conscious, especially when their feet are smelly from being extremely anxious. Then invite them to relax by taking in three long and deep breaths; discourage any further conversation, so that they can drift off into the tranquil alpha state of consciousness and reconnect with their inner self. You are now ready to begin with the warm-up technique (p. 214).

Treat everybody as the most important person in the world.

Helpful reminder

Although it is extremely rewarding to see such amazing results so quickly, remember that, when giving reflexology, you are only a conduit. As such, your role is to encourage the recipient to relax and be more open to receiving universal life force energies, which they can then fully utilize to heal themselves. There is, after all, only one person you can heal and that is yourself!

Rule of thumb

Whether giving reflexology to maintain good health or to help somebody feel better about themselves, always do a complete foot massage, from top to bottom. Pay particular attention to the nervous system and solar plexus reflexes, as well as the endocrine gland and sensory reflexes, while also concentrating on any distressed reflexes. Reflexology is a neutral energy that allows anything that needs to happen, happen!

When first making contact with the recipient, be conscious of how you feel because it sets the tone for the whole session. Although most of the massage is simultaneously on both feet, whenever a sequence involves moving from one foot to the other, always go from the right foot to the left, because the right foot represents the past and the left the present.

10 QUESTIONS TO CONSIDER

1 What's the best way to treat emotional wounds?

2 When it comes to giving reflexology, which are your two most essential tools?

3 How can the most congenial and tranquil healing environment be created?

4 Why should a simple explanation be given to the recipient before starting the treatment?

5 When on medication, when is it best to receive reflexology?

6 How can the recipient be made to feel comfortable?

7 Would you prefer to use powder or oil, or both?

8 Why is conversation, during the treatment, discouraged?

9 Why is it important to understand that it is the recipient who heals themselves?

10 When going from one foot to the other, which foot should ideally be massaged first and why?

10 THINGS TO REMEMBER

1   Everybody has the innate ability to give reflexology.

2   Your own feelings can have a profound effect, both during and after, the massage.

3   Make sure that when giving reflexology, you won't be disturbed by telephones, televisions, family or pets.

4   Use a relaxing chair, bed or sofa for the recipient to lie on and create a relaxing atmosphere with soft, soothing music in the background, appealing aromas and gentle lights to enhance relaxation.

5   Use a stool, chair or cushions to sit comfortably while massaging the feet.

6   Tell the recipient about reflexology, what it is, how it may feel and what to expect afterwards so that they can completely relax and let go.

7   If the recipient is taking prescribed medication, encourage them to tell their doctor of their intention to have reflexology.

8   For those taking medication, the most effective time to give reflexology is an hour before their next dosage, when the body is most receptive and less influenced by the drugs.

9   Remember that although it is very rewarding to see responses and quick results from reflexology, you are only the conduit for the healing to take place.

10 The only person you can truly heal is yourself!

22

Reflexology step by step

In this chapter you will learn:
- *the whole technique*
- *useful tips*
- *what to expect.*

The warm-up

Start the reflexology session by using the caressing movements of the warm-up to encourage the recipient to relax. Take this opportunity to really connect with them and gauge what's going on at a much deeper level. Feel free to adapt any of the following movements to suit their individual needs, as long as it makes them feel safe enough to let go and loosen up, making them more open to receiving and utilizing universal energies.

STEP 1 – CREATE TRUST

Take time to establish a bond so that they feel less vulnerable about baring their soles and their soul to you. To do this, gently take the recipient's heels and rest them lightly in the palms of your hands, either with their feet still covered or uncovered. As you do this, invite them to close their eyes and take in three long, deep breaths (Figure 22.1).

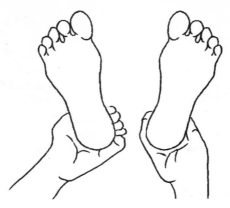

Figure 22.1 Rest their feet in your hands.

STEP 2 – BREATHE AND RELAX

Guide them as they take these breaths, encouraging them to hold each
breath for as long as possible. As they breathe in, suggest they take
in 'pure love' and 'white light' and, as they breathe out, advise them
to let go of anything that no longer serves them. At the same time,
be aware of your own breathing, using it to consciously relax any
tension in your own body, which is generally in the neck, shoulders,
back and upper arms.

At the end of the three deep breaths, ask the recipient to continue
breathing naturally, keeping their eyes closed so that they can focus
inwards. Leave your hands where they are, as you clear your own
mind and reconnect with your spirit, as well as your heart. Take time
to tune into the recipient's energy and be aware of what their body is

'saying'. Don't try to please; just be your wonderful self! Make your mind up to really enjoy every second of however long the session may take. Once starting the massage, constantly vary your pressure from being really gentle but firm, for physical ease, to barely touching the skin's surface, to help lift their spirit. If you believe yourself to be highly sensitive to other people's energies, then encase yourself and the recipient in a beautiful white or pink bubble, so that you each have your own space. Trust your intuition to guide you every step of the way. It's now time for the two of you to experience complete serenity, inner peace and a tremendous boost of life force energy.

> You have brought a special gift to this planet – your unique touch and presence.

Insight

Before the 'warm-up' begins, make it clear that it's time to stop any chitchat so that they can completely let go and relax. Invite them to close their eyes and breathe rhythmically to prevent them from being distracted by the outside world.

STEP 3 – CARESS THE TOPS

Gently lower the recipient's heels onto the bed, then lightly but reassuringly stroke the tops of their feet, hand over hand, towards yourself (Figure 22.2), first on their right foot, then on their left. This is one of the few times that the movements are intentionally

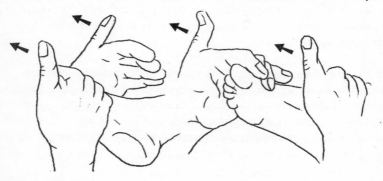

Figure 22.2 Caress the tops.

towards, and not away from, you, because it gives the recipient time to get used to your energy.

STEP 4 – STROKE THEIR SOLES

Next stroke the soles of their right foot, and then of their left foot, with the backs of your hands (Figure 22.3), this time towards the recipient, giving them a little longer to feel comfortable about the position they are in.

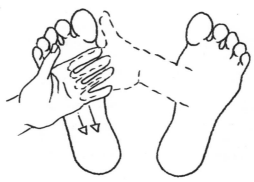

Figure 22.3 Stroke their soles.

Insight

The warm-up sequence embraces mind, body and soul, so both feet are fully embraced. Not only does this indicate that something special has begun, but, by creating trust, it also encourages a greater acceptance of the whole therapeutic process.

STEP 5 – CIRCLE THE ANKLE BONES

With your left fingers resting on the outside and your right fingers on the inside of the right ankle bone, firmly yet sensitively circle around each bone simultaneously (Figure 22.4). Gradually ease your pressure until there is very little or no contact, while, at the same time, steadily removing all your fingers, until only the middle fingers are circling the ankle bones. Repeat on the left foot.

These movements loosen any rigidity in the recipient's approach to life and encourage them to believe more in themselves.

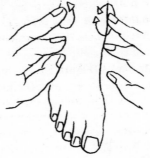

Figure 22.4 Circle the ankle bones.

STEP 6 – SHAKE THE FOOT

Rest the mounds at the bases of both thumbs, in the hollows either side of the recipient's right ankle, just beneath the ankle bones (Figure 22.5). To shake the foot, keep the mounds of your hands in the same position, while moving your one hand towards the recipient and the other, in the opposite direction; then reverse this action. Watch their foot move from side to side, slowly at first, then with greater fervor. Once the right foot has had a good shake, repeat on the left foot. In time, and with practice, you will know whether to speed up or slow down this movement. Effectively loosening the ankles makes it so much easier to adapt to life's ups and downs, as well as be more flexible and forgiving within relationships. It eases the strain of being held back, as well as provides the confidence to stride out and make incredible progress.

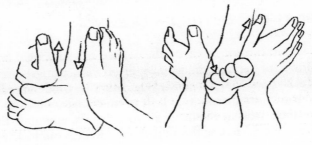

Figure 22.5 Shake the feet.

While doing the warm-up sequence, be aware of how the feet look and feel. Also note whether there are any prominent markings or unusual features. It provides clues as to where special attention is required as the treatment progresses.

STEP 7 – KNEAD DOWNWARDS

Gently rest the balls of the right toes against your right hand or lightly embrace them; make a loose fist with your left hand and place your knuckles just beneath the right toe necks. Knead firmly, but soothingly, all the way down, moving from the outer edge of the right foot to the tips of the heels (Figure 22.6) in a long, steady strip. Repeat from top to bottom, strip by strip, moving across the foot, until reaching the inner edge of the same foot. Now reverse the role of your hands and repeat on the left foot to encourage the recipient to literally 'knuckle down' and get on with making the most of their life, by dealing with the tasks in hand. Opening and clearing the energy pathways assists the recipient in confronting life and doing something worthwhile with their wonderful ideas.

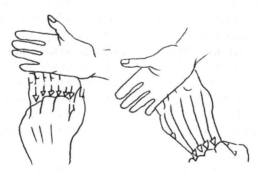

Figure 22.6 Knead downwards.

Insight

Really give the ankles a good shake – they love it! The more flexible they are, the easier it is to relax and become more open to revitalizing energies.

STEP 8 – EXPLORE AND RELEASE

Now place all your fingertips, side by side, on top of the right toes (Figure 22.7) and make tiny circular movements over the top of the right foot, all the way up to the ankle crease; here you separate your two hands so that the fingers can continue massaging either side of their right ankle, to the back of the heels. Repeat the whole procedure three times, reducing your pressure each time, before moving over to their left foot and doing the same. This is a great way of easing any back tension and encouraging the recipient to let go of any unpleasantness that may be going on in the background and holding them back.

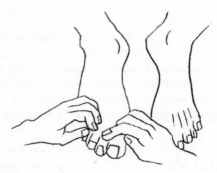

Figure 22.7 Explore and release.

STEP 9 – PULL THE ACHILLES TENDON

For the Achilles pull, the recipient must lie as flat as possible for it to be effective. Place your left hand under their right heel and your right hand on top of the same foot, in alignment with the foot; firmly 'pull' the right heel towards you (Figure 22.8) until a slight resistance is felt, watching the body as it lengthens. Hold the stretch for a short while before very slowly releasing. Repeat this three times, then do the same on their left foot. Not only does this give the legs a good stretch, but it also elongates the spine, releasing any unwanted tension or trapped nerves. By helping the spine realign itself, a free flow of vital life force energies is re-established throughout the body.

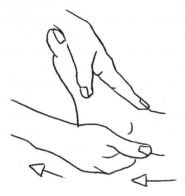

Figure 22.8 Pull the Achilles.

Insight

Firmly embracing and pulling the heels is superb for stretching and extending mind and body. It creates much-needed space between the spinal vertebrae, taking a huge amount of pressure off the nerves. It can be pure bliss!

STEP 10 – STRETCH THE ACHILLES TENDON

Take the recipient's right heel back into your left hand, once again aligning your right hand on top. This time gently, but firmly, bend their right foot downwards (Figure 22.9), stretching the upper surface as far as possible without resistance. Hold this stretch for a short while before allowing the foot to slowly return to its natural position. Repeat three times and then do the same on the left foot. The purpose is to create greater awareness of when to hold back

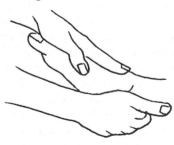

Figure 22.9 Stretch the foot.

and when to step forwards, while remaining open to the possibility of being stretched from time to time. This movement can be alternated with the Achilles pull for a more fluid action.

STEP 11 – RUB THE SPINAL REFLEXES

Use the heel of your right hand to caress the bony arch (Figure 22.10), first on the right foot, moving from the big toe to the ankle bone. Apply slight pressure as your hand eases its way up to the ankle bone, then lightly and slowly drag your hand back to their big toe. Repeat this a few times, before doing the same on their left arch, this time, using the heel of your left hand. This is an excellent way of calming the nerves, getting rid of inappropriate beliefs and encouraging complete relaxation.

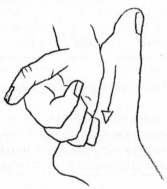

Figure 22.10 Rub the spinal reflexes.

> **Insight**
> While rubbing the spinal reflexes, feel their shape and mentally note any conspicuous lumps and bumps since these indicate areas where additional support is being sought and reached out for.

IN BETWEEN SEQUENCES

In between each sequence, cup both hands over the toes on the right foot, with your fingers on the top and thumbs underneath;

then, with a loving squeeze, move your hands, simultaneously towards the ankles; now separate your hands so that they cup the feet and then caress upwards on either side of the feet (Figure 22.11). Do this at least three times before repeating it on the left foot. This is a caring way of creating overall harmony, accelerating the healing process and reassuring the recipient. It's also a very effective way of warming cold feet.

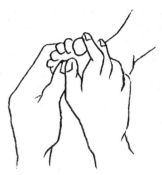

Figure 22.11 In between sequences.

Insight

The gentle, overall massage of the feet between each section of a treatment defines the beginning and end of a sequence. It also provides time to adjust and tune into the varying energies of the next system that is to be massaged.

Soothe the nerves

Always massage the nervous system reflexes first because the brain controls the functioning of the whole body. With the mind calm, the recipient is relieved of any fear or anxiety and their body can relax. Also by balancing the intellect and the intuition, the recipient has greater insight into what really satisfies their soul so that their journey through life is more meaningful and manageable.

STEP 12 – OPEN THE ENERGY FLOWS

Begin by opening the energy flows to ensure that the mind is more receptive to the healing. Gently place all your fingertips onto the tips of each of the corresponding toes, except for the big toes (Figure 22.12). Apply gentle pressure, hold for a few seconds, and then gradually ease the pressure until your fingertips are just resting or hovering above the toe surfaces.

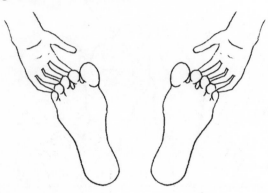

Figure 22.12 Open the energy flows 1.

> ### Insight
> If any of the toes, especially the big toes, lean to the side, use your fingers to straighten them. This not only makes them look better but allows the energies to flow more freely. It brings the mind into the present and encourages the soul to realign itself.

Remove your fingers and lightly place the tips of your thumbs onto the tips of each big toe (Figure 22.13). Again apply slight pressure for a few seconds before gradually easing off, until your thumbs rest lightly or hover marginally above the big toes. To enhance the effect, mentally infuse the toes with ether, while visualizing indigo, violet, purple and/or white. This will help to open up the energy flows even more. Overused and outdated beliefs can then escape, taking with them any fearful notions or frightful memories.

You may notice the body jerking and twitching as energy reaches parts that it hasn't been able to access for some time. You may also feel a delightful tingling or intense heat between your fingers and the recipient's toes; a sign that healing is actively taking place. This is a truly amazing way of reconnecting with the universal energies and of encouraging the recipient to link with their true spirit for greater compassion towards themselves and the whole of humanity. After all, at soul level, we are 'all one'.

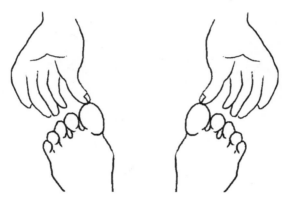

Figure 22.13 Open the energy flows 2.

STEP 13 – EASE THE MIND

Simultaneously, rest your little fingers on the tips of the outer edges of the little toes (Figure 22.14). Gently push down for a few seconds, then ease off, lightly rotating your digits (p. 194) at the same time. Move your fingers fractionally along the tips of the little toes and repeat this pumping and rotating movement. Continue until the tops of both little toes have been well stimulated. Now place your ring fingers onto the outer edges of the tips of the fourth toes and do the same; repeat with your middle fingers on the third toes; then with your index fingers on the second toes and finally your thumbs on the big toes. Return your little fingers to the outer edges of the little toes but, this time, place them slightly lower down; continue the technique all the way across all of the toe pads, from the little to the big toes, starting a fraction lower down each time until the toe pads have been thoroughly massaged. This takes a weight off the mind, improves brain activity, expands the capacity to think, makes more space for exciting new concepts, prolongs concentration and favourably alters thought patterns. Furthermore, by calming or exciting the hypothalamus, at the base of the brain, it affects the production and functioning of hormones, for even greater inner harmony. Ultimately a healthier state of mind ensures a much healthier and happier body.

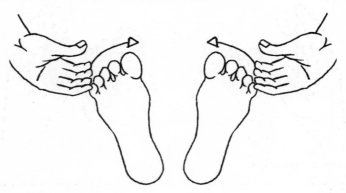

Figure 22.14 Ease the mind.

STEP 14 – REJUVENATE THE FACE

To rejuvenate the face repeat the above sequence but this time, place your thumbs on the recipient's little toe pads, with the little finger directly opposite, on the upper surfaces; to substantially increase the energy flow. Should the vibration be too intense for the recipient, then lift the supporting fingers while maintaining contact with your thumbs only. Repeat on each pair of toes, simultaneously, using the corresponding fingers on the upper surfaces. Once all the toes have been thoroughly massaged (Figure 22.15), milk them one by one (p. 195), going from the right to the left foot, starting at the tips of each toe and milking down to their bases, from the outer to the inner edges; now feather caress (p. 196) each toe using the same sequence. Spend additional time on 'congested' reflexes and massage the big toes particularly well since the main brain and sensory reflexes are here.

The idea is to boost self-confidence, making it that much easier to face the world as an individual.

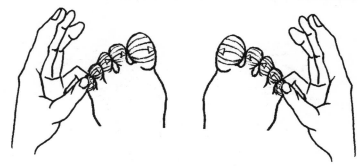

Figure 22.15 Rejuvenate the face.

STEP 15 – IMPROVE THE EYESIGHT

Place your thumbs over the centres of both little toe pads, with your little fingers directly opposite, on the upper surfaces of the little toes (Figure 22.16). Lightly squeeze the two digits together until a slight resistance is felt; hold for a few seconds then gently and slowly rotate your thumbs, while visualizing red. Gradually ease the pressure until there is little or no contact. Now lightly rest your little fingers on the hubs of the toe pads, over the eye reflexes, for a short while. Repeat the procedure on the mounds of the fourth toe pads, this time using your thumbs with your ring fingers, while visualizing orange; then do the same on the mounds of the third toes, with your thumbs and middle fingers, with yellow in mind; then on the mounds of the second toes with your thumbs and index fingers, picturing green and, finally, on the hubs of the big toe pads, with your thumbs on the toe pads and your index fingers on top, imagining purple and blue. This technique is ideal for improving eyesight, sharpening vision, easing eye strain, broadening the outlook, clarifying perceptions, helping to focus better, maximizing optical functioning and balancing the recipient's interpretation of what's going on in their emotional environment.

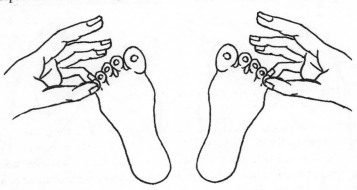

Figure 22.16 Improve the eyesight.

Insight

All toe pads reflect the ears, nose, eyes and mouth, so the massage helps to fine-tune the sensory system. It clears emotional blockages that may have been interfering with the ability to hear, see, smell or taste, which makes it possible to, once again, get in touch with true meaning.

STEP 16 – ACKNOWLEDGE THE NOSE

Place your thumbs on the nose reflexes, on the inner joints of both big toes (Figure 22.17), with your middle fingers providing support on the opposite side. Gradually press the thumbs in, rotate them gently and then release. Now replace the thumbs with your middle fingers and rest them on these reflexes for a few seconds, visualizing yellow to enhance the sense of smell and encourage self-recognition. Acknowledging the nose is a way of ensuring that the recipient is on track and doing what they should be doing. The massage further helps them to find their way by 'following their nose'.

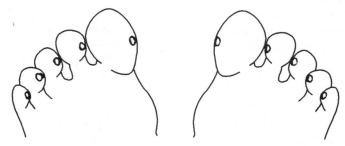

Figure 22.17 Acknowledge the nose.

STEP 17 – FOR BETTER HEARING

To massage the ear reflexes, place your middle fingers on the outer joints of the recipient's little toes, over the ear reflexes (Figure 22.18), using your thumbs to support from the other side. If using the middle fingers is too awkward, then replace them with your little fingers. Press and rotate (p. 194) with your fingers, for a few seconds, then gently squeeze the two digits together before lightly, but firmly, milking both sides simultaneously, from top to bottom, applying a slight amount of compression between the two digits. Repeat over the ear reflexes on the fourth toes, using your ring fingers with your thumbs supporting; then go on to the third toes, using your middle fingers supporting with your thumbs; move on to the second toes, using your index fingers with your thumbs

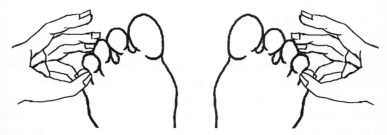

Figure 22.18 For better hearing.

supporting; and, finally, on to the big toes, but this time place your thumbs over the ear reflexes and use your middle fingers to support. Stimulating the ear reflexes enhances hearing, improves listening skills, creates awareness of the inner mind chatter, makes sounds clearer and clarifies their meaning, increases alertness, improves balance and assists in the accurate interpretation of all that is heard.

STEP 18 – SOOTHE THE MOUTH

Position your thumbs on the mouth reflexes (Figure 22.19), just beneath the inner joints of both big toes, placing your ring fingers on the opposite sides for support. Gradually press your thumbs in, then gently rotate before slowly releasing. Now place the tips of your ring fingers on both mouth reflexes for a few seconds, visualizing orange, to facilitate speech, ease decision making, enhance self-confidence and for greater belief in personal concepts.

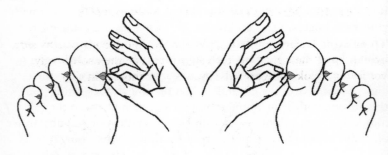

Figure 22.19 Soothe the mouth.

STEP 19 – RELAX THE JAW

Massage the jaw reflexes (Figure 22.20) using the rotation technique at the bases of each pair of toe pads simultaneously to ease tension and prevent the grinding of teeth. This will also increase mobility, as well as confidence to ensure that innovative ideas are shared with greater conviction.

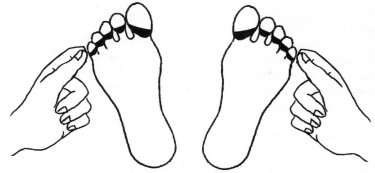

Figure 22.20 Relax the jaw.

Insight

The jaw becomes tense from words that have been left unsaid, while the teeth are affected by decision making. Together they determine the amount of flexibility in the jaw, which, in turn, affects the ability to 'chew things over'.

STEP 20 – MILK THE FACIAL LYMPHATICS

To milk the facial lymphatics, place your thumb pads side by side on the tip of the right little toe (Figure 22.21), then soothingly, yet firmly, stroke downwards, thumb over thumb, in tiny

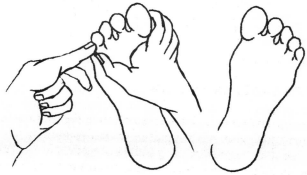

Figure 22.21 Milk the facial lymphatics.

movements, from top to bottom. Do this several times until the right little toe pad is thoroughly milked. Now do the same on the fourth right toe, followed by the middle right toe, then the second right toe and eventually the big right toe. Repeat the whole procedure, in exactly the same way, on the left toes, starting with the little left toe. This helps in easing mental congestion and deeply ingrained impressions. In so doing, it clears the old to make way for the new, in the hope of opening the recipient's mind to every point of view.

STEP 21 – OVER THE BACK OF THE HEAD AND NECK

To massage the back of the head and neck, place all your fingers on the outer edges of the little toes, either side of the recipient's feet. 'Walk' them in unison over the upper surfaces of all the toes (Figure 22.22), finishing on the inner edges of both big toes. Repeat a few times for the recipient to clear the clutter at the back of their mind, to evacuate fearful memories from their deep subconscious, to strengthen belief in themselves and to provide a firm backing for their own ideas.

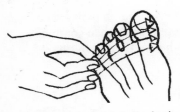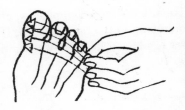

Figure 22.22 Over the back of the head and neck.

Insight

The upper surfaces of all toes reflect the back of the mind; their appearance is influenced by all the mental clutter that is crammed in. Hair or corns appear when thoughts, hovering in the background, are being concealed or protected.

Open the avenues of expression

STEP 22 – CLEAR THE THROAT

Place your thumbs onto the recipient's little toe necks, with your middle fingers on the other side (Figure 22.23). Gently squeeze the two digits together, hold for a while then gradually release while, at the same time, lightly rotating (p. 194) with your thumbs, until there is little or no contact. Now do the same on the fourth toe necks with the thumbs and ring fingers; on the third toe necks with the thumbs and middle fingers; on the second toe necks with the thumbs and index fingers, finishing on the big toe necks.

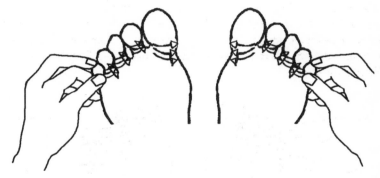

Figure 22.23 Clear the throat.

Insight

Any form of expression that enters or leaves the body determines the direction and impact of energy. So ask yourself whether you are speaking up. If not, why not? Is there anybody who is being a pain in the neck? Who is it? Which aspects of you are they mirroring? Are you willing to see every point of view?

STEP 23 – CARESS THE NECK

Use your thumbs to gently, but firmly, stroke and milk the underneath surfaces of all toe necks, from top to bottom (Figure 22.24). Start on the right toe necks, going from the little to the big toe necks, then do the same on the left toe necks. Give additional attention to the sides, where there's often a lot of tension, due to unresolved emotions that remain unexpressed. Next feather stroke each toe neck, from the right little toe neck to the right big toe neck, then the left little toe neck to the left big toe neck. It effectively eases neck and throat tension, assists lymph activity and increases blood flow to and from the head, opening up all the main avenues of self-expression.

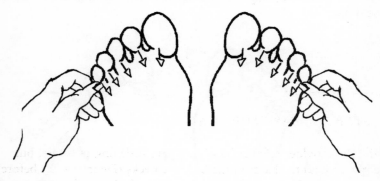

Figure 22.24 Caress the neck.

Insight

The more relaxed the neck, the greater its mobility and potential for glimpsing opportunities. Being flexible makes it easier to see every point of view and expand the mind. So it is that 'milking' the toe necks thoroughly opens up the avenue of expression, encouraging stored emotions to be trustingly brought up.

STEP 24 – WEIGHT OFF THE SHOULDERS

To massage the shoulder reflexes, position your thumbs on the outer edges of the balls of both feet, immediately beneath the recipient's little toe necks, resting your middle fingers, directly opposite, on the tops of the little toe necks (Figure 22.25). Lightly squeeze the two together then gently rotate (p. 194) your thumbs. Glide the digits along the ridge, immediately beneath the toe necks, repeating the movement below each toe up to the big toe necks. Repeat several times, especially if these reflexes feel hard and swollen or lack substance.

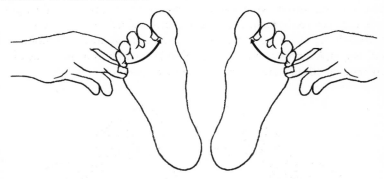

Figure 22.25 A weight off the shoulders.

STEP 25 – EASE THE LOAD

Milk the shoulder reflexes by sliding your little fingers firmly, but gently, around the bases of the little toe necks (Figure 22.26) before slipping them through the gaps between the little and fourth toes; bring your little fingers back again, then glide them around the

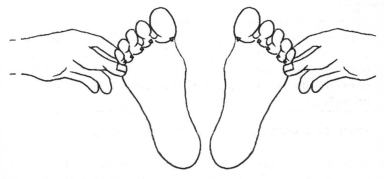

Figure 22.26 Ease the load.

bases of the fourth toe necks before slithering them through the gaps between the fourth and third toes. Keep doing this through all the gaps between the toes and repeat up to three times to take a 'weight off the shoulders', to ease the need to 'shoulder responsibilities', to allow all the 'shoulds' and 'shouldn'ts' to slip away and to enhance the flow of life force energies to the head, specifically to the ears and eyes. Since this also relaxes the clavicle bones, the chest can expand, improving the stature.

Insight

Heart energies travel via the shoulders to the arms where they become evident through hugging and touching. Shoulder issues arise from conflicting emotions, a fear of intimacy, hurt at being rejected, or when putting other's needs first. The shoulders become rigid, which stagnates the energies and blocks the flow. Reflexology assists in releasing hefty emotional burdens that weigh them down.

STEP 26 – RELEASE NECK TENSION

To release tension at the back of the neck, place all your fingers either side of the recipient's toe necks (Figure 22.27) and 'walk' them, in unison, over the tops of all the toe necks, as far as the inner edges of the big toe necks. Repeat this movement two to three more times before milking. Now lightly run all your fingers, from the tips of the toes, over the tops of the feet, to the ankle creases. All in all, these caresses help to increase neck flexibility, creating greater harmony between the recipient's internal and external environments.

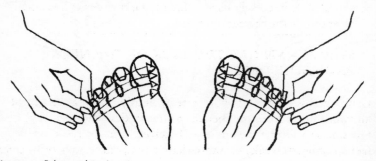

Figure 22.27 Release neck tension.

STEP 27 – BALANCE THE MIND

Lightly rest your middle fingers onto the tips of both little toes (Figure 22.28), leave them there for a few seconds before moving on to the joints of the toes; stay for a while then place them at the bases of both little toes. Repeat these three balancing touches on the upper surfaces of the fourth toes, then the third toes, followed by the second toes and finally the big toes, to help centre the mind and put everything into perspective.

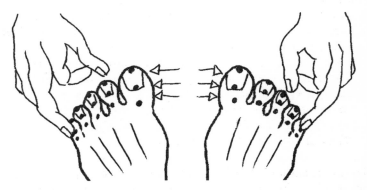

Figure 22.28 Balance the mind.

Insight

The brain is the body's computer; whatever is put into it determines the type of outcome, based on programmed beliefs and stored memories. Outdated notions can be deleted by massaging the toes, which then makes space for a vital shift in consciousness. Balancing the toes calms and harmonizes the thought process.

STEP 28 – STROKE THE BACK OF THE NECK AND SHOULDERS

Gently caress the tops of both feet by lightly running the tips of all your fingers from the toenails to the ankles (Figure 22.29) a few times to soothe the anxiety of 'getting it in the neck' or of feeling obliged to take on more than is really necessary or to clear anything hurtful or upsetting going on in the background.

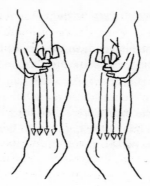

Figure 22.29 Soothing the nerves.

Re-establish a firm backbone

STEP 29 – CO-ORDINATE MIND AND BODY

To massage the midbrain reflexes, place your thumbs or fingers on the tips of both big toes (Figure 22.30) and gently massage down their inner edges, as far as their joints; repeat by moving the digit a fraction to the top and then to the bottom of the strip making sure that the small area is thoroughly massaged. Now milk with tiny

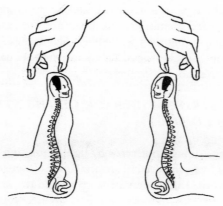

Figure 22.30 Co-ordinate mind and body.

soothing strokes and then lightly feather. Doing this co-ordinates mind and body, fine-tunes muscular co-ordination, improves respiration, enhances cardiac and circulatory functioning and encourages a more balanced approach to life.

Insight

The arches of the insteps provide a natural, elastic spring to the step when walking, jumping, dancing and so on. This also prevents any jarring, which, in turn, protects the spine, which they so clearly reflect. Once the nerves are calmed, through massage, then the spine can easily convey harmonious messages from the brain to the rest of the body.

STEP 30 – ENSURE A FIRM BACKING

To strengthen the spine, place your thumbs or fingers on the inner joints of both big toes (Figure 22.31) and gently massage, with rotation or caterpillar movements, along the complete length of the bony ridges that border the insides of the recipient's feet. Finish just beneath the inner ankle bones; then repeat, but this time angle your thumbs downwards, so that they are angled onto the tops of the bony ridges. Massaging the length of this ridge stimulates or calms the sensory nerves. Do this again, but, this time, with your thumbs gently pushing upwards, underneath the bony ridges, so that the

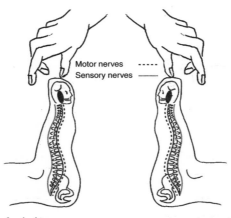

Figure 22.31 Ensure a firm backing.

motor nerves are accessed. Follow by milking first the right spinal reflex, with small, repetitive soothing strokes, from the big toe to the ankle, and then the left spinal reflex in the same way. Complete the sequence with an exceptionally light feathering, also from top to bottom, which either soothes agitated nerves or stimulates petrified nerves. All cells benefit from these caresses because of the nerves radiating from the spinal cord and infiltrating the whole body. Massaging the spinal reflexes facilitates the relay of nervous messages, while, at the same time, increases each cell's awareness of its environment. This enables mind and body to function at their best.

Insight

In the 1960s, Robert St. John was so disillusioned at the tendency to revert back to illness and disease that he channelled through an ancient technique, known as the 'Metamorphic Technique'. It's based on the idea that because the spine is in constant contact with the womb, the unborn baby is constantly aware of its mother's thoughts and feelings.

STEP 31 – EASE THE NECK

Repeat step 30, from the joints of the big toes to their bases (Figure 22.32), particularly for neck problems, so that flexibility is increased for every point of view to be clearly seen.

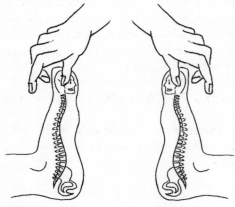

Figure 22.32 Ease the neck.

STEP 32 – CARESS THE UPPER BACK

Repeat step 30, but now go along the inner edges of both balls of the feet (Figure 22.33), to boost emotional backing and support, as well as provide greater emotional strength.

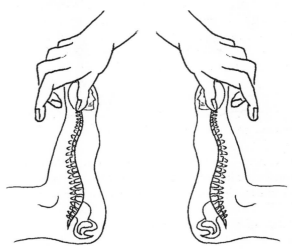

Figure 22.33 Caress the upper back.

Insight

The upper back is where memories of hurt feelings, along with those of fear, guilt, shame and emotional confusion are stored; it's also where lost desires are deeply buried. Visualizing green, whilst massaging these reflexes, helps to re-establish emotional support.

STEP 33 – STRENGTHEN THE UPPER MIDDLE BACK

Repeat step 30, from the bases of the balls of the feet to both waistlines of the feet (Figure 22.34), for the strength to keep going, no matter what!

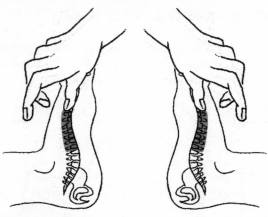

Figure 22.34 Strengthen the upper middle back.

> **Insight**
>
> The upper middle back is where memories of what was done or not done reside. They are generally filled with frustration and resentment at having felt so spineless, helpless or powerless. Whilst massaging these reflexes, visualize yellow to throw light on these situations and become self-supportive.

STEP 34 – REASSURE THE LOWER MIDDLE BACK

Repeat step 30, from the waistlines of both feet to the junctions where the insteps and heels meet (Figure 22.35), for sound relationships and greater backup in all forms of communication.

> **Insight**
>
> The middle back gets caught between personal needs and the requirements of others, while the lower middle back tends to hang on to the memories of those who have been unceremoniously shoved into the background. Visualizing orange, whilst massaging these reflexes, assists in resolving unresolved issues and provides the compassion to finally let go.

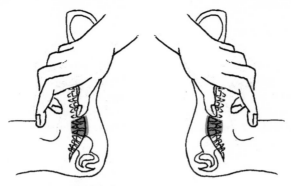

Figure 22.35 Reassure the lower middle back.

STEP 35 – EMPOWER THE LOWER BACK

Repeat step 30, around the bases of the inner ankles (Figure 22.36), to ease lower back pain through the re-establishment of self-empowerment and greater inner resourcefulness.

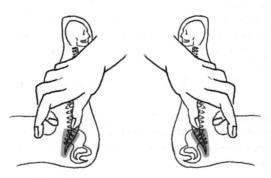

Figure 22.36 Empower the lower back.

Insight

The lower back can be a real pain when there's insufficient family and social support or not enough financial backing. This anguish can spread down the legs to the feet and cause numbness. It's a good time to 'see red', whilst massaging these reflexes, since it's a colour filled with a lot of energy and potential!

The metamorphic technique

The metamorphic technique completes the spinal reflexes procedure by effectively liberating past fears and anxieties, particularly those experienced while in the womb. The tips of the big toes signify the time of conception, the spinal reflexes reflect the time in the womb, while the ends of the bony ridges, just beneath both inner ankles, represent the time of birth (Figure 22.37).

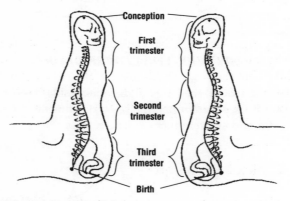

Figure 22.37 Reflections of time in the womb.

Insight

When massaging the spinal reflexes, take it one step further; use each corresponding pair of digits over the relevant spinal reflexes. Start with the thumbs on the big toes, change to the second fingers over the edges of the balls of the feet, use the middle fingers as far as the 'waistline' of the spine, then the ring fingers to the bases of the arches, finishing with the little fingers under the inner ankle bones.

STEP 36 – RELEASE THE PAST

Lightly place the tips of your middle fingers onto the tips of the big toes; these points represent the time of conception. Visualize a beautiful white light, as you take three long deep breaths.

Keep your fingers still for a few seconds, then, barely touching the skin's surface, glide them slowly along the spinal reflexes, to where they end just below the inner ankles, which symbolize the time of birth. Leave your fingers here for a while and, again, visualize a bright white light. Repeat the whole sequence another two to three times. For one or two of the sequences, try using tiny circular movements, instead of just gliding. This powerful technique effectively cuts the invisible umbilical cord between the recipient and their mother, freeing them both of the need to be caught up in each other's energy. It allows them to be their own unique selves.

Insight

Allow any digits to instinctively fall onto the tips of each big toe at the start of the metamorphic technique; they could well differ, but this is great! They draw attention to areas of concern and are ideal for providing the remedy required for any issues still outstanding since the time in the womb.

The solar plexus technique

The solar plexus reflexes are the most powerful on the feet and can be massaged at any time to calm the recipient, should they panic for any reason.

STEP 37 – CREATE A CENTRE OF CALM

Place both thumbs on the hollows (Figure 22.38) immediately beneath the balls of the feet and apply a gentle, but firm, pressure until a slight resistance is felt. Keep your thumbs still for a while and then gradually ease off, until the tips of your thumbs barely touch the skin's surface. Lightly stroke the reflexes either with your thumbs or middle fingers, before resting the tips of either digit on the hollows for a few seconds. This immediately creates an inner calm. It can also relieve asthmatic attacks and bronchial spasms, soothe palpitations, reduce hysteria and regulate hyperventilation. Massaging these reflexes induces an incredible sense of serenity and peace throughout.

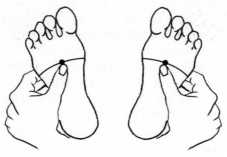

Figure 22.38 Create a centre of calm.

Insight

While massaging the solar plexus reflexes, be conscious
that they are the doorway to the innermost being. Notice
how far your thumbs can venture inwards before there's a
resistance; also detect whether there is any difference
between the right (past) and left (present) solar plexus
reflexes.

Harmonize the endocrine system

The endocrine reflexes are generally quite sensitive, especially
when there's a related issue. Always massage these reflexes
immediately after the nervous system reflexes since they rely on
the hypothalamus, at the base of the brain, as well as the nerves,
to provide the information required to function well.

STEP 38 – OPEN THE ENERGY FLOW

First open the energy flows (Figures 22.39 and 22.40), as explained
in step 12, to make the glands more receptive to receiving the
universal energies.

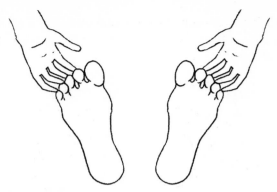

Figure 22.39 Open the energy flow.

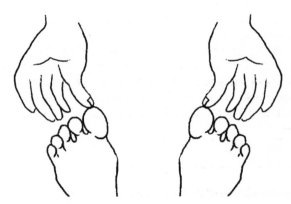

Figure 22.40 Opening the energy flow.

STEP 39 – PUT THE PITUITARY GLAND BACK IN CONTROL

To help the pituitary gland function well, lightly drop your thumbs onto the upper ledges of the inner joints of both big toes (Figure 22.41). Apply gentle pressure, while gyrating your thumbs at the same time; then hold your thumbs still for a while before gradually easing off the pressure. Now place the tips of your middle fingers on these reflexes and lightly rest them here for a few seconds, while visualizing violet for greater clarity. This also calms the emotions, creates inner harmony and balances the hormonal secretions, all of which improves the overall functioning of all the endocrine glands.

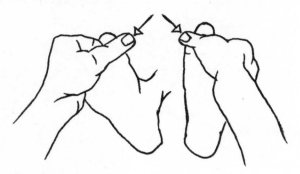

Figure 22.41 Put the pituitary gland in control.

Insight

See the pituitary gland as the conductor of the endocrine orchestra. When leading the way in harmonious and perfect time, the other hormonal glands will naturally follow!

STEP 40 – GREATER INSIGHT THROUGH THE PINEAL GLAND

To stimulate the pineal gland, place your thumbs on the central mounds of both big toe pads (Figure 22.42) with your index fingers placed directly opposite. Squeeze the two digits gently together and then gradually release, while rotating with the thumbs. Now remove your thumbs. Lightly rest the tips of your index fingers in their place, onto the eye reflexes, and visualize indigo to harmonize the natural cycle, regulate the menstrual cycle, stabilize mood swings, enhance intuition and enlighten mind, body and soul.

Insight

Stimulating the pineal gland reflexes augments insight. For revelations around the family and society, rest the thumbs onto the centres of the little toe pads; for relationships, onto the fourth toe pads; for decisions about what to do or not do, onto the third toe pads; for innermost feelings, onto the second toe pads and finally for insight into core beliefs, onto the centres of the big toe.

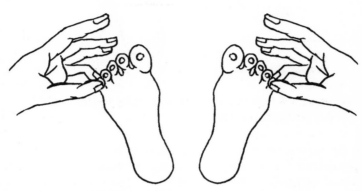

Figure 22.42 Gain insight through the pineal gland.

STEP 41 – MAKE SPACE FOR THE THYROID GLAND

To massage the thyroid gland, lightly place your thumbs on the inner edges of the creases, at the bases of the big toes (Figure 22.43). Gently press down, hold for a while, and then, as you ease the pressure, lightly rotate. Replace your thumbs with the tips of your index fingers; resting them here for a short while and visualizing an exquisite turquoise blue. Now soothingly stroke the thyroid reflexes with your index fingers, to reduce the anxiety of constantly trying to get on top of situations and for balance to be restored. Once the metabolism is working well, the recipient is able to just be themselves.

Insight

The butterfly-shaped thyroid gland represents transformation into becoming one's true self. Massaging its reflexes can assist in creating much needed space to 'spread the wings and fly'.

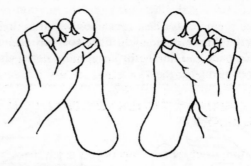

Figure 22.43 Make space for the thyroid gland.

STEP 42 – RECONNECT WITH THE SPIRIT VIA THE THYMUS GLAND

For the recipient to reconnect with their authentic self, feel for slight indentations or possible swellings, halfway down the inner edges of both balls of the recipient's feet. Rest your thumbs here, with your index fingers positioned directly opposite (Figure 22.44). Now gently squeeze the digits together and hold for a few seconds. As you ease the pressure, slowly rotate your thumbs; replace them with your index fingers, slowly resting them on the thymus gland reflexes, while visualizing green; then lightly stroke with these fingers. Reconnecting with the spirit through the thymus gland reflexes encourages the recipient to really believe in themselves and, in so doing, boosts their immunity.

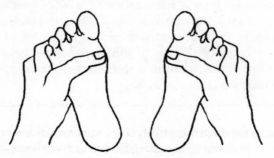

Figure 22.44 Reconnect with the spirit via the thymus gland.

STEP 43 – FINDING COURAGE THROUGH THE ADRENALS

Place your thumbs or middle fingers on the adrenal gland reflexes (Figure 22.45), with your right digit slightly further in and fractionally lower down than your left. Apply minimal pressure and hold briefly before releasing while, at the same time, using the rotation technique. Gently milk with your thumbs; then feather caress with your middle fingers; now lightly rest the tips of these fingers on the adrenal gland reflexes for a few seconds, visualizing yellow to enhance the effect. This puts the recipient at ease and gives them the courage to implement their extraordinary and often unbelievable concepts, no matter what others say or think. It makes the seemingly impossible possible.

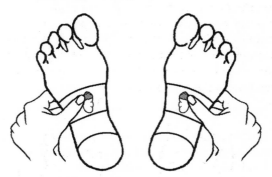

Figure 22.45 Find courage through the adrenal glands.

STEP 44 – GENERATE NEW CONCEPTS THROUGH THE OVARIES

Massage the ovary reflexes on both genders since everybody has male and female energies. Place your thumbs or ring fingers on the ovary reflexes (Figure 22.46), apply slight pressure, hold for a while, then gradually ease off while, at the same time, gently rotating your digits. Lightly stroke the reflexes, then rest your ring fingers on them for a few seconds, visualizing orange. Generating new concepts, via the ovarian reflexes, encourages the recipient to connect with their creative juices, as well as their gentler, more sensitive feminine qualities.

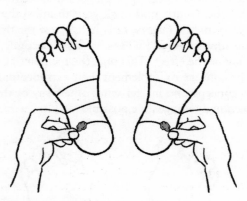

Figure 22.46 Generate new concepts through the ovaries.

Insight

The secondary reflexes for the ovaries are shared by the two high stress indentations, found above the buttocks, and are situated, on both feet, in the hollows between the outer ankle bones and tips of the heels. They are, therefore, likely to be highly sensitive.

STEP 45 – TEST THE WAY WITH THE TESTES

The testes reflexes are also massaged on both genders because of the male and female energies being present in everybody. You may need to feel around the inner heels to find the testes reflexes, since they tend to move. Once you have found them, place your thumbs or little fingers on their reflexes (Figure 22.47), press down slightly and then, as you ease off, gently massage. Milk lightly with your thumbs; then feather with your little fingers, while visualizing red. This ensures that the testes test the way and make a worthwhile contribution to the betterment and advancement of humankind.

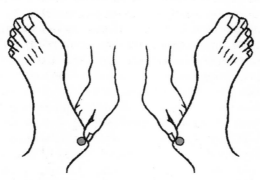

Figure 22.47 Test the way with the testes.

Insight

The testes store ancestral memories and knowledge, passed on from father to son. Honouring the important contribution men make to society helps in harmonizing the mind, body and soul. When it comes to reflexology, the testes reflexes are massaged on both males and females to acknowledge forefathers and resolve any outstanding issues.

It's time, once again, for the 'in-between' sequence, detailed on p. 222, so embrace each foot and lightly 'squeeze' from the tips of the toes to the ankles and heels to enhance the overall effect of massaging the nervous and endocrine reflexes.

Take in the breath of life

The respiratory and cardiac system reflexes are massaged next to help the recipient to become reacquainted with their true spirit through the breath of life. Since these areas are linked to self-esteem and self-worth, massaging them also helps the recipient feel better about themselves and others.

STEP 46 – EXPAND THE LUNGS

For the lungs to expand, place your thumbs, immediately beneath the shoulder reflexes, on the outer edges of the balls of both feet, with your index fingers directly opposite (Figure 22.48). Gently, but firmly, squeeze the two digits together and then slowly release, while lightly rotating your thumbs. Horizontally move both digits fractionally along and keep doing this, across the balls of the feet, to the bases of the big toes; now take your digits back to the outer edges, but, this time, place them a fraction lower down and massage the next horizontal strip. Continue doing this, strip by strip, all the way down until both balls of the feet have been thoroughly massaged. It expands the lung reflexes and ensures that there is plenty of space in which to breathe, allowing the recipient to adapt, more effortlessly, to the constant emotional changes within their environment.

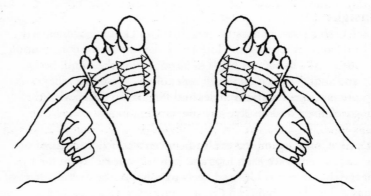

Figure 22.48 Expand the lungs.

Insight

When massaging the lung reflexes on the balls of the feet, watch the recipient's breath, since they often take in deep breaths as the heaviness lifts off their chests.

STEP 47 – TAKE IT ALL IN

Once again, place your thumbs onto the balls of both feet, just below the little toes (Figure 22.49) and then either caterpillar or rotate downwards in vertical strips, from top to bottom, until both balls of the feet have been completely massaged. Now go to the outer edges of the right foot and milk firmly downwards, thumb over thumb, also in vertical strips, moving from the outside to the inside. Then, very lightly feather caress, in the same way, with your index fingers. Repeat on the ball of the left foot.

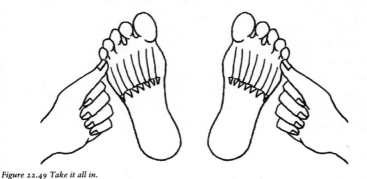

Figure 22.49 Take it all in.

STEP 48 – KEEP ABREAST

The breasts are automatically caressed at the same time as the lung reflexes (Figure 22.50), easing any emotional congestion. Massaging the breast reflexes facilitates the nurturing process and creates more harmonious internal and external environments.

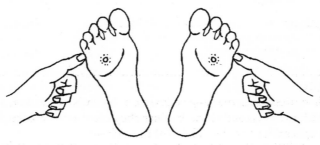

Figure 22.50 Keep abreast.

STEP 49 – RENEW THE LOVE IN THE HEART

To renew the love in the heart, lightly place the tips of your index and middle fingers over the heart reflexes (Figure 22.51) on the inner edges, where the balls of the feet and insteps come together. Apply slight pressure for a while and then gradually ease off while gently rotating the digits. Rest for a moment before lovingly stroking these sensitive reflexes, while visualizing green or pink to enhance the effect. Renewing the love in the heart strengthens and purifies the recipient's affections and opens their heart to even greater love for themselves and others. Wherever there's love, there is health.

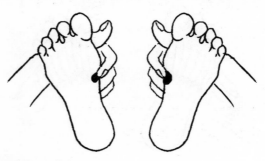

Figure 22.51 Renew the love in the heart.

Insight
When massaging the heart reflexes, open your own heart to love. As the energy of love enters you, it will naturally channel through to the recipient.

STEP 50 – FIRM UP THE RIBCAGE

To massage the ribcage reflexes, place all your fingers either side of the balls of both feet. 'Walk' them several times, in unison, across the tops of both feet (Figure 22.52) from the outer to the inner edges; then, using the heels of your hands, gently caress the upper surfaces, this time going up the feet from the toes to the ankles. Finish by lightly running all your fingers in the same direction. The idea is to encourage the recipient to find the inner strength to emotionally back themselves.

Once again, it's time for the 'in-between' sequence, detailed on p. 222, during which you fully embrace each foot and 'hug' it, from the toes to the heels, enhancing the overall effect of massaging the respiratory and cardiac systems, as well as breast reflexes.

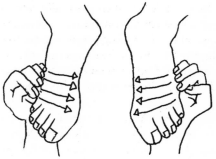

Figure 22.52 Firm up the ribcage.

Restore the digestive system

There are two parts to the digestive system; the accessory organs, which include the liver, pancreas and spleen, all of which aid digestion, according to what happened in the past, and then there's the digestive tract itself, which processes things as they happen in the here and now. Massage the accessory organ reflexes first, to sort things out, especially after a rough patch; the organs are then in a better condition to assist in dealing with the present.

Insight

The liver, pancreas and spleen reflexes are all massaged before the alimentary canal reflexes, since they play such a vital role in assisting the digestive process, analysing past events. They are well positioned to provide the input required to digest current circumstances.

STEP 51 – ENLIVEN THE LIVER

Stimulate the liver reflexes (Figure 22.53) by placing your left thumb on the outer edge of the right sole instep, immediately beneath the ball of the right foot, and your right thumb, a fraction lower down, on the opposite edge of the same foot. Either caterpillar or rotate your left thumb, horizontally across the sole instep, from the recipient's right to their left, all the way to your right thumb. Place your left thumb back at the starting point but, this time, a little lower down, then keep it still as you massage towards it with your right thumb, from the inner to the outer edges of the right sole instep. Continue alternating the digits and massaging in both directions until the whole triangular reflex of the liver is thoroughly massaged. Now milk firmly downwards, thumb over thumb. Finish by lightly caressing the whole reflex with your third and ring fingers, from top to bottom. Although a tiny portion of the liver is also reflected onto the left foot, this is massaged at the same time as the left stomach reflex (p. 263), so it requires no specific action, unless you feel that it needs it. Enlivening the liver reflexes helps in sorting out past events and provides ample energy in the present. It also gives the recipient the impetus to implement their own ideas for personal growth and development. Massaging these reflexes ensures that a consistent and favourable temperature is maintained throughout the body.

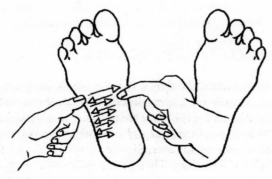

Figure 22.53 Enliven the liver.

STEP 52 – HAVE THE GALL

To massage the gall bladder reflex (Figure 22.54), rest your left thumb or third finger midway along the lower triangular edge of the liver reflex, on the right foot only. Gently rotate your digit on this minuscule ball-like reflex, then milk thumb over thumb in a downward movement, on the same spot, and then lightly feather with your middle fingers. Massaging these reflexes dissipates resentment and bitterness, making it possible to move on with peace of mind.

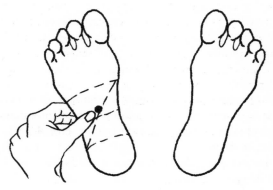

Figure 22.54 Have the gall.

STEP 53 – PLEASE THE PANCREAS

To soothe the pancreatic reflexes, rest the whole length of your left thumb across the foot, immediately beneath the waistline of the recipient's left foot; keep it there to use as a guideline (Figure 22.55). Now place your right thumb at the tip of this tadpole-shaped reflex and caterpillar or rotate your digit from the recipient's left to their right. Then firmly milk, thumb over thumb, across the reflex in the same direction, before lightly feathering downwards with your middle fingers. Now move over to the right foot, once again placing the whole length of your left thumb across the right foot immediately beneath the waistline and repeat the same procedure, still moving from the recipient's right to their left, as far as the centre of the foot. This balances the pancreas and creates an inner peace about all that is taking place.

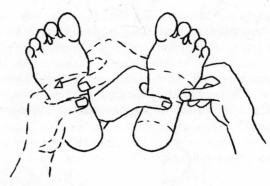

Figure 22.55 Please the pancreas.

STEP 54 – SURPRISE THE SPLEEN

With your thumbs either side of the spleen reflex (Figure 22.56), on the upper, outer quadrant of the recipient's left fleshy instep, gently caterpillar or rotate in both directions until the whole reflex has been thoroughly massaged. Then firmly milk downwards, thumb over thumb, before lightly feathering with your middle fingers. This encourages the recipient to have a balanced approach to life, in all that they do for themselves and others.

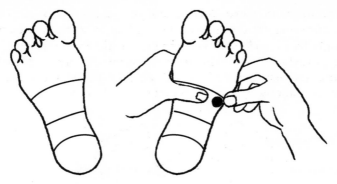

Figure 22.56 Surprise the spleen.

It's time once again for the 'in-between massage', detailed on p. 222, so lovingly embrace each foot, from top to bottom, to enhance the overall effect of massaging the liver, gall bladder, pancreas and spleen reflexes.

Re-energize the whole system

Next the digestive tract itself is massaged from the mouth reflexes, on the big toes, to the anal reflexes, on the inner heels, since the bulk of the digestive organ reflexes are reflected onto the sole insteps.

Insight

When massaging the digestive tract, visualize the anatomical journey that the food makes from the mouth to the anus and follow this when going through the sequence of movements.

STEP 55 – IN THE MOUTH

Place your thumbs or ring fingers on the mouth reflexes (Figure 22.57), just below the joints of the big toes; apply slight pressure and gently rotate. Appeasing the mouth reflexes facilitates the chewing process, improves the sense of taste and assists with decision making.

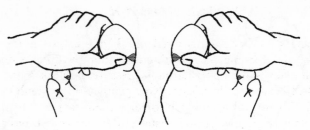

Figure 22.57 In the mouth.

STEP 56 – SOOTHE THE OESOPHAGUS

Soothe the oesophagus reflexes (Figure 22.58) by caterpillaring or rotating, with your thumbs or index fingers, from the mouth reflexes, along the throat reflexes and then all the way down the inner edges of the balls of both feet. Do this several times before lightly milking with your thumbs. Finish by gently feather stroking with your index fingers, to pacify or excite the peristaltic action. Soothing the oesophagus reflexes assists with taking in and swallowing the fullness of life's experiences with far greater understanding.

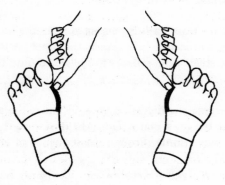

Figure 22.58 Soothe the oesophagus.

Insight
Visualizing green, when massaging along the oesophagus reflexes, helps to calm any choking emotions, making it easier to swallow unpalatable situations.

STEP 57 – OPEN THE STOMACH

Massage the cardiac sphincter reflexes (Figure 22.59), at the entrance of the stomach, by resting your thumbs or index fingers on both reflexes and applying slight pressure; hold for a few seconds, then gradually release. Now gently stroke thumb over thumb. This opens the stomach to being more receptive to all that comes its way, no matter how distasteful it may sometimes seem.

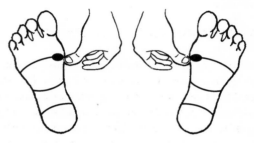

Figure 22.59 Open the stomach.

Insight

While massaging the stomach reflexes visualize how food is churned and mimic these actions; it assists in the effective 'breakdown' of food, which then eases it onto the next stage of digestion.

STEP 58 – RUB THE TUMMY

Visualize the stomach reflex in the upper, inner quadrant of the left foot (Figure 22.60) then, using either the caterpillar or rotation technique, massage it horizontally, either with your thumbs or middle fingers, go from one side of the reflex to the other to mimic the churning movement of the stomach. Next milk horizontally, thumb over thumb, towards the right foot, before feathering in the same direction, with your middle fingers. Now massage the small portion of stomach reflex on the right foot, this time going from the recipient's left to their right. Rubbing the tummy reflexes assists in 'stomaching' life's ongoing experiences and reinforces the ability to cope, no matter what!

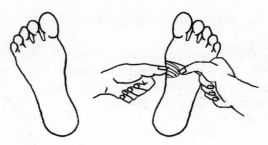

Figure 22.60 Rub the tummy.

STEP 59 – MOVE IT ON

At the exit of the stomach is the pyloric sphincter. Massage this reflex (Figure 22.61) by applying slight pressure, then hold for a few seconds, before slowly releasing and lightly massaging with your middle fingers. Palpating the pyloric sphincter reflexes helps the recipient in moving on to the next stage of their life.

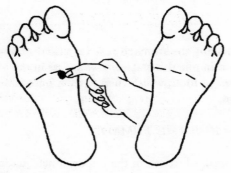

Figure 22.61 Move it on.

STEP 60 – AROUND THE 'C' OF THE DUODENUM

Use your right thumb to massage the C-shaped duodenum reflex, only on the inner, upper quadrant of the right foot (Figure 22.62). Either use the rotation or caterpillar movement, changing your thumbs midway to make the movement flow better. Then lightly milk the 'C' before gently feathering with your middle fingers. Going around the 'C' of the duodenum reflex helps the recipient to finish dealing with past issues so that they can get on and enjoy the present.

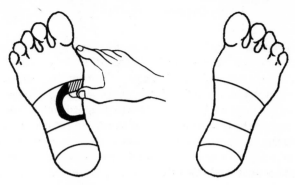

Figure 22.62 Around the 'C' of the duodenum.

Insight

To release upsetting memories that 'eat away' at the insides, visualize yellow while massaging the duodenum reflex, since memories tend to have an impact on what's going on.

STEP 61 – CAJOLE THE JEJUNUM

Massage the jejunum reflex (Figure 22.63), just above or on the waistline of the left foot, moving from the recipient's right to their left. Now gently milk this short reflex, thumb over thumb, in the same direction, before lightly feathering with your middle fingers. Cajoling the jejunum reflex persuades the recipient to take the next exciting step and keep things moving.

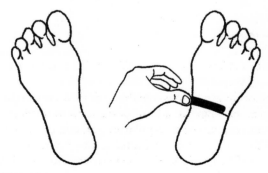

Figure 22.63 Cajole the jejunum.

STEP 62 – WIND THROUGH THE SMALL INTESTINES

Wind through the small intestines by placing your right thumb or right ring finger at the start of the small intestine reflex (Figure 22.64), then massage horizontally from the recipient's left to their right, using the base of the waistline as a guideline. Go from their left foot and continue on their right foot. At the outer edge of their right foot, use your left thumb to return across both insteps in the opposite direction, immediately beneath the previous horizontal strip. Continue, backwards and forwards, from one side to the other, until both lower sole insteps have been thoroughly massaged. Now lightly milk with your thumbs, in the same way, then gently feather stroke the whole area with your ring fingers. Winding through the small intestine reflexes assists in establishing greater tolerance and understanding within relationships.

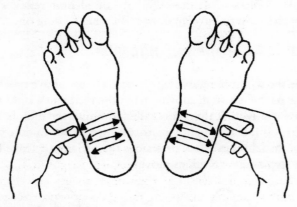

Figure 22.64 Wind through the small intestines.

Insight

The small intestines take the best out of situations, leaving the wasteful aspects, which are moved on to the large colon to be expelled from the body. Massage these reflexes to encourage a more balanced give and take in relationships.

STEP 63 – REASSURE THE ILEO-CAECAL VALVE

Place your right thumb or middle finger on the ileo-caecal valve reflex (Figure 22.65), in the lower, outer corner of the right fleshy instep. Apply slight pressure, hold for a while, then gradually release, while gently rotating. Now lightly stroke the reflex with your ring fingers. Reassuring the ileo-caecal valve reflex helps in getting rid of the old to make way for the new.

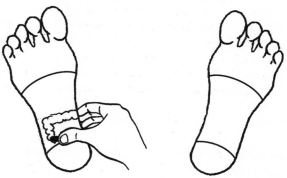

Figure 22.65 Reassure the ileo-caecal valve.

STEP 64 – CLEAR OUT THE APPENDIX

Place your left thumb or fourth finger on the appendix reflex (Figure 22.66), found only on the recipient's right foot. Massage this minuscule reflex with tiny rotational movements, then lightly stroke with your ring fingers. Agitating the appendix reflex helps those who feel that their life is going nowhere, along with those caught up in a dead-end relationship or job.

Insight

Even if the appendix has been removed, its energy remains; massage its reflex to avoid the consequences of being in a dead-end relationship.

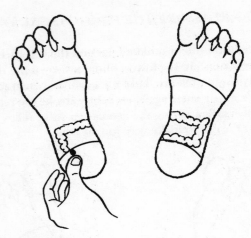

Figure 22.66 Clear out the appendix.

STEP 65 – UP THE ASCENDING COLON

Place your left thumb at the base of the ascending colon reflex (Figure 22.67) and massage up the reflex, as far as the waistline, then milk it firmly with both thumbs. Now lightly feather stroke with your ring fingers. Going up the ascending colon facilitates the onward movement of remnants from what was done or not done, that would otherwise waste time and energy.

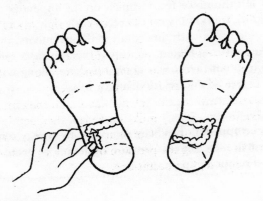

Figure 22.67 Up the ascending colon.

STEP 66 – AROUND THE HEPATIC FLEXURE

Feel for a swelling on or just below the waistline (Figure 22.68) of the right foot. Apply slight pressure, hold it for a while and then release. Now turn the digit so that it points towards the left foot. It helps the recipient to turn corners with greater ease.

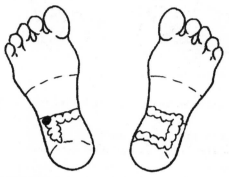

Figure 22.68 Around the hepatic flexure.

Insight

Always use forward movements when following the reflexes of the large colon, to ensure that wastes don't get stuck or blocked on their way to being evacuated.

STEP 67 – ACROSS THE TRANSVERSE COLON

Massage the transverse colon reflexes (Figure 22.69), following the base of the waistline, from the hepatic flexure reflex on the right foot to the centre of the left foot; here you need to massage very slightly upwards, towards the splenic flexure on the outer edge of the left sole instep. Firmly milk this reflex, then gently feather stroke with your ring fingers. Going across the transverse colon reflexes helps in relieving the pressure of having to perform and meet unreasonably high expectations.

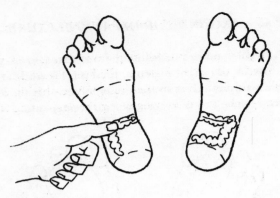

Figure 22.69 Across the transverse colon.

STEP 68 – AROUND THE SPLENIC FLEXURE

With your left thumb, feel for the slight swelling of the splenic flexure reflex (Figure 22.70) and massage it well. Now turn your right thumb so that it's angled downwards and apply slight pressure. Hold for a while and then release. Massaging the splenic reflex prevents hiccups getting in the way.

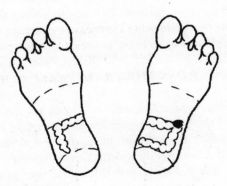

Figure 22.70 Around the splenic flexure.

> ### Insight
> Massage the hepatic, splenic and sigmoid flexures really well to ensure that no wastes or unwanted remnants get caught up in awkward situations or tricky corners.

STEP 69 – DOWN THE DESCENDING COLON

With your right thumb, still pointing downwards, massage down the outer border of the left instep to the heel (Figure 22.71), then firmly milk with both thumbs, before lightly feathering with your ring fingers, to get wastes moving along the descending colon.

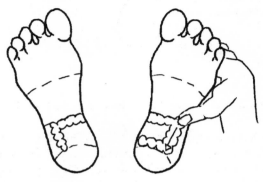

Figure 22.71 Down the descending colon.

STEP 70 – SKIRT THE SIGMOID FLEXURE

Rest your right thumb on the sigmoid flexure reflex, in the lower corner of the left sole instep (Figure 22.72), and apply slight pressure. Hold this for a while and then release. Now turn your thumb so that it's pointing towards the inside edge of the left foot.

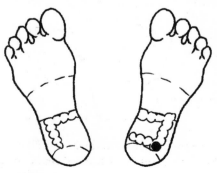

Figure 22.72 Skirt the sigmoid flexure.

STEP 71 – SLITHER ALONG THE SIGMOID COLON

Slither your right thumb along the sigmoid colon reflex, at the base of the left sole instep, just above the heel pad, going from the recipient's left to their right (Figure 22.73). Now firmly milk, thumb over thumb, before lightly feathering with your ring fingers. Slithering along the sigmoid colon reflexes keeps remnants moving and helps them on their way out.

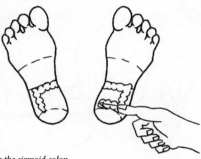

Figure 22.73 Slither along the sigmoid colon.

STEP 72 – OUT THROUGH THE RECTUM

Massage the arcs of the rectum reflexes by placing your thumbs or little fingers on the inner edges of both feet, at the junction where the heels and insteps meet (Figure 22.74), by either caterpillaring or rotating. Now firmly milk, thumb over thumb, then gently feather stroke with the little fingers. Stimulating the rectum reflexes eases the release of all the rough aspects of life.

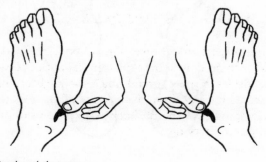

Figure 22.74 Out through the rectum.

STEP 73 – ANGLING FOR THE ANUS

Apply slight pressure to the anus reflexes (Figure 22.75), hold it for a few seconds, and now release. Next firmly stroke these reflexes with your thumbs, then caress lightly with your little fingers. Agitating the anus reflexes forces the recipient to experience the utter relief of totally letting go and, in so doing, complete the digestive process.

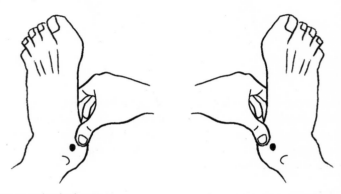

Figure 22.75 Angling for the anus.

Insight

It's tempting to get bogged down by the past but it feels so much better to move on from nasty memories! Although challenging, it's the only way to make space for exciting new energy and experiences. Massage the rectum and anus reflexes well to assist this natural flow.

STEP 74 – OVER THE MIDDLE BACK

Place all your fingers on the outer edges of both insteps (Figure 22.76) and 'walk' them in unison over the tops, from the outsides of the feet to the insides. Repeat several times, then lightly run the tips of your fingers up the feet, from the bases of all the toes to the ankle creases. Going over the middle back reflexes helps to provide the inner strength to carry on.

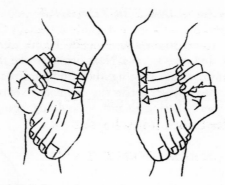

Figure 22.76 Over the middle back.

Insight

The energy of countless memories, of what happened or didn't happen, reside in the background, so spend time massaging the tops of both feet, as well as the inner edges of the insteps. This helps to evict any dreadful memories, takes pressure off the back and allows it to strengthen itself.

STEP 75 – SOOTHING THE INNARDS

Use all your fingers to walk along the fleshy insteps on the inner edges of the feet (Figure 22.77), immediately below the bony arch. Now milk, with the heels of your hands, moving towards the recipient; finally, run all your fingers along these reflexes. Soothing the innards ensures ongoing resourcefulness.

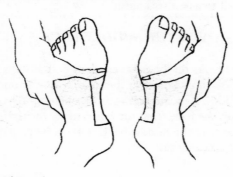

Figure 22.77 Soothing the innards.

It's time for the in-between sequence again, detailed on p. 222, so lovingly embrace each foot and gently squeeze it from top to bottom, to enhance the overall effect of the digestive procedure.

Reinstate the bones, muscles and skin

STEP 76 – STRENGTHEN THE PELVIS

Place your thumbs or little fingers onto the outer edges of both heel pads, where they join the insteps (Figure 22.78) and firmly massage in horizontal strips, from the outer to the inner edges of both heels, either by caterpillaring or rotating. Keep repeating this, moving your digits fractionally down each time, until both heels have been thoroughly massaged. Next milk downwards, thumb over thumb, from the outer to the inner edges, then lightly feather stroke with your little fingers. Strengthening the pelvic reflexes helps in providing a solid foundation, as well as greater mobility and flexibility, especially during childbirth.

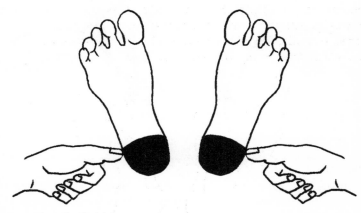

Figure 22.78 Strengthen the pelvis.

Do the in-between sequence again, as detailed on p. 222,
embracing each foot and lightly squeezing it, from top to bottom,
to enhance the overall effect of massaging the pelvic reflexes.

Restrengthen the limbs

STEP 77 – ALONG THE UPPER ARM REFLEXES

Place your thumbs or index fingers immediately below the little
toes and simultaneously massage along the outer edges of the balls
of both feet (Figure 22.79) to the elbow reflexes. Now firmly milk,
thumb over thumb, and then feather caress with your little fingers.
Massaging the upper arm reflexes provides the confidence to reach
out and embrace new beginnings.

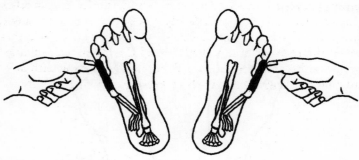

Figure 22.79 Along the upper arm reflexes.

STEP 78 – FLEX THE ELBOWS

Generously use the rotation technique on the elbow reflexes (Figure 22.80), which are the prominent bones midway down the outer edges of both feet; then firmly milk them, before lightly feathering, with your second and middle fingers, to give the recipient room to be themselves.

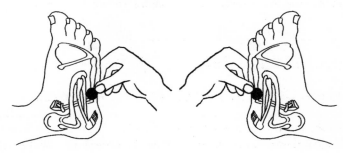

Figure 22.80 Flex the elbows.

STEP 79 – DOWN THE LOWER ARM

Use your thumbs, or middle fingers, to massage the lower arm reflexes (Figure 22.81), along the outside edges of both feet at a 45° angle, between the elbow and hand reflexes. Now firmly milk along these reflexes, thumb over thumb, then caress lightly with your middle fingers. Soothing the lower arm reflexes helps in coping with any emotional challenges that have been kept 'at arm's length'.

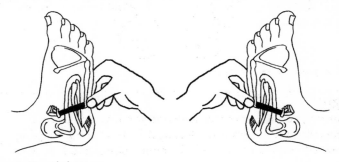

Figure 22.81 Down the lower arm.

STEP 80 – TEND TO THE HANDS

Tend to the hands (Figure 22.82) in the same way as the elbow reflexes (step 78), to facilitate the handling of the many aspects of life.

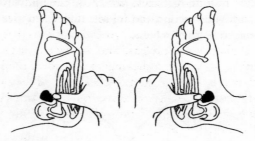

Figure 22.82 Tend to the hands.

Insight

The hand reflexes either swell when overwhelmed from handling so much, or become insignificant and sink when withdrawing and not wishing to get involved. Either way, they love the helping hand of reflexology.

STEP 81 – UP THE THIGHS

To massage the reflexes for the thighs (Figure 22.83), place your thumbs or ring fingers on the knee reflexes, then caterpillar or rotate your digits up towards the base of the outer ankle bones. Now milk with both thumbs, then stroke lightly with your ring fingers. Massaging the thigh reflexes helps in being more open to life's opportunities and to move on when necessary.

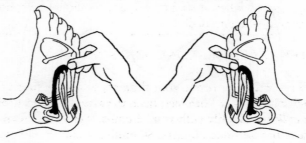

Figure 22.83 Up the thighs.

STEP 82 – KNEAD THE KNEES

Place your thumbs on the recipient's shoulder reflexes and your middle fingers on their elbow reflexes, then use your index fingers to feel for the tiny bony ledges, just above the midway point between the two reflexes; these are secondary accesses to the knees (Figure 22.84). Now place your thumbs on these reflexes and apply slight pressure, release and massage thoroughly, then stroke lightly with your middle fingers. Kneading the knee reflexes encourages the recipient to be more flexible and to adapt more easily to unexpected changes of direction. The primary reflexes, for the knees, are stimulated when massaging the nipple reflexes on the balls of the feet (p. 255).

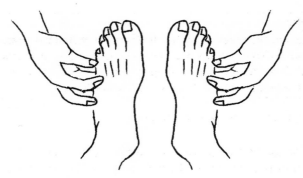

Figure 22.84 Knead the knees.

Insight

Visualizing green while massaging the knee reflexes releases any rigidity, when stuck in a rut, and facilitates a change in direction when needed.

STEP 83 – SKIM ALONG THE SHINS

Either caterpillar or rotate your thumbs, or middle fingers, along the outer borders of both feet, from the knee to the feet reflexes. Now milk thoroughly with your thumbs, then gently feather stroke with your index fingers. Skimming along the shin reflexes

(Figure 22.85) provides greater scope and strength, especially when it comes to following through with certain activities.

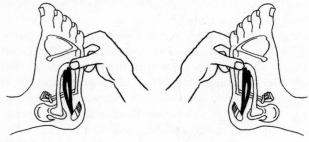

Figure 22.85 Skim along the shins.

STEP 84 – EMBRACE THE FEET

Massage the foot reflexes (Figure 22.86) by rotating your thumbs, then stroking and feathering to provide even greater stability and mobility.

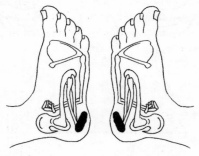

Figure 22.86 Embrace the feet.

Insight

Even the feet have reflexes on the feet! Massaging these areas provides the impetus to get going.

STEP 85 – BOLSTER THE BUTTOCKS

Caress the buttock reflexes (Figure 22.87) on the outer triangular areas of both heels either with your thumbs or all your fingers; do this several times. Then soothe these areas with the heels of your hands, before lightly feathering with all your fingers. Bolstering the buttock reflexes helps strengthen the seat of power.

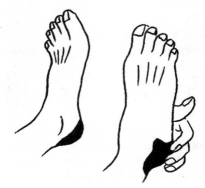

Figure 22.87 Bolster the buttocks.

STEP 86 – REINFORCE THE HIPS

Circle around the hip reflexes (Figure 22.88), on the outer ankle bones, several times, with either your thumbs or all your fingers, first firmly, then lightly, to provide the impetus and force needed to move ahead with ease.

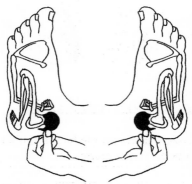

Figure 22.88 Reinforce the hips.

Appease the reproductive organs

STEP 87 – ATTEND TO THE FALLOPIAN TUBES

Place your thumbs or ring fingers on the ovary reflexes (Figure 22.89) and massage from the outer to the inner aspects of the lower fleshy insteps, with gentle rotation movements. Next lightly milk thumb over thumb, then gently feather stroke with your ring fingers, to clear the way for new ideas to come through.

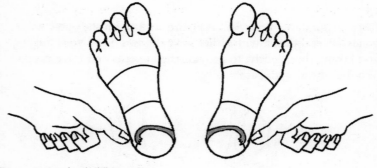

Figure 22.89 Attend to the fallopian tubes.

STEP 88 – FROM THE OTHER SIDE

Now massage the secondary fallopian tube reflexes from the other side (Figure 22.90) this time by caterpillaring, then milking, from the outer to the inner ankle bones, along the ankle creases, to further assist in bringing new concepts out into the open.

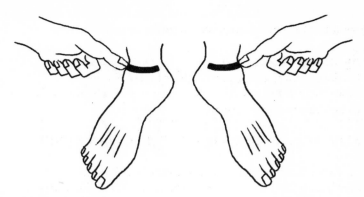

Figure 22.90 From the other side.

STEP 89 – UNLEASH THE UTERUS

Gently massage the uterus reflexes (Figure 22.91) with your thumbs or little fingers, then lightly stroke and caress them, especially during pregnancy, to create a more harmonious environment within the home, as well as balance the feminine energy.

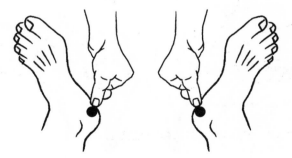

Figure 22.91 Unleash the uterus.

STEP 90 – SOOTHE THE VAGINA

Soothe the vaginal reflexes (Figure 22.92), by rotating either with your thumbs or little fingers on the slight indentations on the insides, midway between the ankle bone and heels; then lightly stroke and caress them, to encourage a much gentler approach to life.

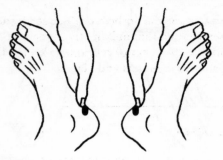

Figure 22.92 Soothe the vagina.

STEP 91 – BOLSTER MANLY ASSETS

Thoroughly massage the inner triangular areas on both heels, either with your thumbs or with all of your fingers; now milk well, then feather with your little fingers. Bolstering the male reproductive reflexes (Figure 22.93) improves inner strength, enhances personal performance and makes the recipient feel important, so that they can rise appropriately to any occasion.

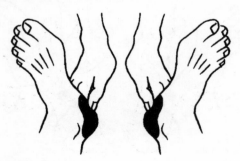

Figure 22.93 Bolster manly assets.

Insight

The inner heels hold the reproductive reflexes for both male and female. They are synonymous with new concepts in the mind, the courage to bring them to fruition and the ability to do something worthwhile with them.

It's time once again for the 'in-between' sequence, detailed on p. 222, so embrace each foot and lightly squeeze it, from top to bottom, to enhance the effect of reflexology on the limb, buttock and lower reproductive organs and glands.

Release the past

STEP 92 – WORK THROUGH THE KIDNEYS

Place your thumbs, or ring fingers, pointing downwards, at the top of both kidney reflexes (Figure 22.94) and massage the tiny strips of about an inch, from top to bottom, either by caterpillaring or rotating your digits. Next milk thoroughly with your thumbs, then feather stroke with your middle and ring fingers. Massaging the kidney reflexes helps to eliminate worked-through and outdated thoughts and emotions, thereby encouraging a harmonious environment for the ideal balance within relationships.

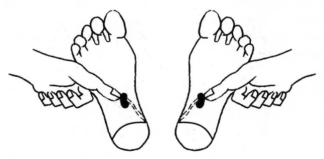

Figure 22.94 Work through the kidneys.

Insight

Massaging the kidney reflexes encourages them to filter out thoughts and emotions that have been processed and are now ready for release.

STEP 93 – SQUEEZE THE URETERS

To milk the ureter reflexes, place your thumbs or ring fingers halfway along the kidney reflexes (Figure 22.95) and caterpillar or rotate down to the bladder reflexes. Now milk with your thumbs, then feather stroke with your ring fingers.

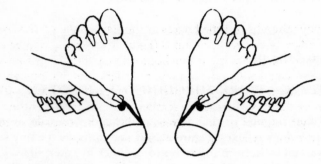

Figure 22.95 Squeeze the ureters.

STEP 94 – REASSURE THE BLADDER

Rest your thumbs or little fingers on the fleshy mounds at the bases of the inner heels (Figure 22.96) and gently palpate these reflexes. Now lightly milk them, and then tenderly feather stroke them with your little fingers. Reassuring the bladder makes it so much more accommodating.

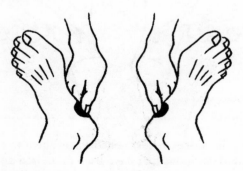

Figure 22.96 Reassure the bladder.

STEP 95 – AID THE FLOW

Place your thumbs or little fingers at the start of the urethra reflexes
on the edges of the fleshy mounds (Figures 22.97 and 22.98) and
massage to the tips of the inside heels on men and to the midway
hollow on women. Concentrate on the slight indentations on
females and on the tips of the heels on males. Now firmly milk
with your thumbs, then gently feather stroke with your little
fingers. Massaging the urethral reflexes helps the recipient regain
inner control, especially during distressing periods.

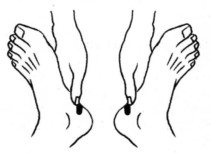

Figure 22.97 Aid the flow on females.

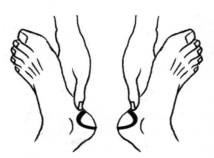

Figure 22.98 Aid the flow on males.

Now do the in-between sequence, detailed on p. 222, by embracing each foot and lightly squeezing it, from top to bottom, to enhance the overall effect of massaging the excretory system.

The finale

By this time, the recipient should be completely relaxed, making it an ideal opportunity to gently stretch and extend the feet for greater flexibility and expansion of mind, body and soul.

STEP 96 – STRETCH THE MIND AND SPINE

Gently pull both little toes simultaneously (Figure 22.99) then release; now pull the fourth toes and let go; do the same on the third toes, the second toes and finally the big toes. Gently tug the big toes for slightly longer. This is an excellent way to relieve neck tension, headaches, back disorders, as well as encourage the recipient to open up to all those possibilities that are available to them.

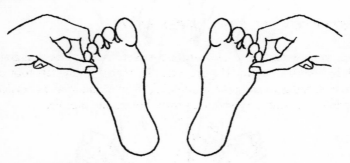

Figure 22.99 Stretch the mind and spine.

> **Insight**
> Once the whole treatment is finished, relax into the finale, encouraging the feet to stretch and loosen up so that any last remnants of tension can be eased.

STEP 97 – EXTEND THE NECK

Lightly support the base of the right little toe, between your left thumb and index finger, then take the right little toe between your right thumb and index finger and rotate it, first anti-clockwise and then clockwise (Figure 22.100). Do the same with the fourth right toe, and then with each toe, one by one. Now repeat on the left foot, starting with the left little toe and finishing with the left big toe. Spend extra time on rotating both big toes since it effectively eases neck tension and loosens up mind and body.

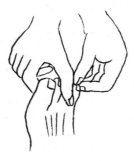

Figure 22.100 Extend the neck.

STEP 98 – FLEX THE UPPER BODY

Place your hands either side of the recipient's right foot and gently roll it from side to side (Figure 22.101); repeat on the left foot to facilitate the give and take in life and, in so doing, make it easier to expand and contract, which, in turn, boosts the morale.

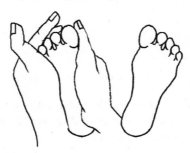

Figure 22.101 Flex the upper body.

STEP 99 – EXTEND THE WHOLE BEING

With both hands on top of the recipient's feet, gently, but firmly, stretch the feet downwards, hold for a while (Figure 22.102) and then release. Next place the palms of your hands flat against both soles and coax the feet upwards. This simple technique is great for broadening horizons and encourages a more amenable approach to life.

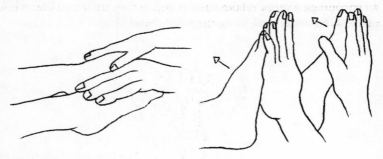

Figure 22.102 Extend the whole being.

STEP 100 – RELAX THE LOWER TORSO

Support the right heel with your left hand and use your right hand to rotate the right foot, as fully as possible, first anti-clockwise and then clockwise (Figure 22.103). Change hands and repeat on the left foot. This relaxes the lower torso, balancing the odds and keeping life events in proportion.

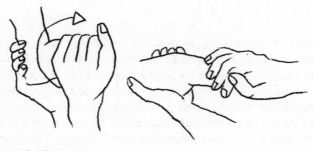

Figure 22.103 Relax the lower torso.

STEP 101 – LOOSEN UP

Place your thumbs together, immediately beneath the right middle toe neck, with your fingers resting on top (Figure 22.104); then gently push up with your thumbs, while using your fingers to lightly stretch the top of the foot over the soles. Repeat this several times, as your hands gradually progress all the way down the middle portion of the right foot. Now do the same on the left foot, to encourage a more relaxed and contented approach to life, while, at the same time, energizing the whole being.

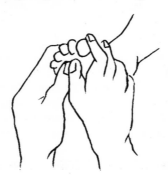

Figure 22.104 Loosen up.

Insight

Allow your hands to flow and guide you through the finale. Also, this is the opportunity to try out some different massage moves.

STEP 102 – THE FINAL STEP

Complete the reflexology sequence by massaging the solar plexus reflexes for a minute or two. Place your thumbs on the hollows (Figure 22.105), immediately beneath the balls of the feet, and apply gentle pressure until a slight resistance is felt. Keep your thumbs still for a while, then slowly ease off, until the tips of your thumbs barely touch the skin's surface. Now lightly stroke the reflexes, either with your thumbs or middle fingers, then rest the tips of your middle fingers on the hollows for a few seconds.

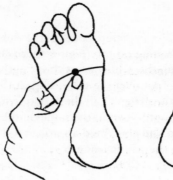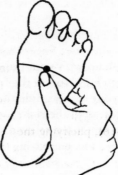

Figure 22.105 The final step.

STEP 103 – BRINGING THE SESSION TO AN END

Stroke first the right foot, from top to bottom, and then the left foot in the same way. Cover both feet, and then continue to hold the covered feet for a little longer. As you do so, use a soft voice to invite the recipient to take in three deep breaths, before opening their eyes, so that they can begin to surface in their own time. A glass of water helps to ground them, as well as flush out their system and enhance the effect of having their feet massaged, which is why they should continue to drink plenty of water. Also suggest that they wrap up well, especially if it's cold outside, since a tremendous amount of heat can be lost, during and after a treatment, because of being so relaxed.

First-aid reflexology

Ideally always give a complete massage on both feet to ensure overall wellbeing through homeostasis of mind, body and soul. Occasionally, however, when there is insufficient time, giving a quick massage is better than nothing. This entails massaging all the toes thoroughly (steps 12–28), soothing the spinal reflexes (steps 29–36), pacifying the solar plexus reflexes (step 37) and balancing the energy centres (steps 38–45). Always finish with the 'in between' massage (p. 222) of both feet. Should there be a particular discomfort in the body, massage its related reflex or reflexes as well. End the short massage by soothing the solar plexus reflexes (step 37).

If you are at all concerned

If, at any time, you are at all concerned, or the recipient panics for any reason, then immediately place your thumbs on their solar plexus reflexes and ask them to take in long, deep breaths. Guide them into relaxing more and more with each out breath, reassuring them that the reaction is only temporary and it's a good sign that a favourable shift has taken place. If it's available, also give them a few drops of rescue remedy.

Insight
Before the recipient leaves tell them that the effects of the reflexology will continue for some time; remind them that any after-effects are a sign that the body is responding well!

10 QUESTIONS TO CONSIDER

1 Why are both feet simultaneously massaged when giving reflexology?

2 Why does the treatment start at the tips of the toes and gradually progress down the feet?

3 What is the role of the warm-up sequence?

4 How are the energy channels of the body and soul opened and re-energized via the feet?

5 Why are the feet caressed and stroked all over between each sequence?

6 Which are the first and most essential reflexes that need to be focused on?

7 Describe the sequence, step by step.

8 Draw your own feet on a piece of paper and then draw in the various reflexes to help you visualize them.

9 Why are the kidneys, bladder and lymphatic reflexes caressed towards the end of the treatment?

10 How is the session brought to a close and why should the recipient take three deep breaths before moving?

10 THINGS TO REMEMBER

1 *When doing the Universal approach to reflexology, both feet are massaged simultaneously, systematically going through each major system's reflexes, from the toes down.*

2 *The warm-up technique is used to 'tune in' to the recipient's energies via the feet.*

3 *Open up the channels with white light and pure love, by resting your fingers on the tips of the toes.*

4 *In between each sequence, lovingly embrace each foot three times to calm, yet accentuate the healing.*

5 *Focus first on the central nervous system reflexes (toes), spinal reflexes (inner bony ridges), solar plexus reflexes (indentations under the ball of the foot) and the endocrine gland reflexes (specific points throughout the feet).*

6 *Next the reflexes for the shoulders (strips along base of all toe necks), the chest and lungs (balls of feet) as well as the heart (inner lower edge of the balls of the feet) reflexes are massaged.*

7 *After this the reflexes for the liver, gall bladder, spleen and pancreas are given attention, followed by the entire digestive process, from the mouth to the anus, the bulk of which are in the sole insteps.*

8 *Following on after this are the reflexes for the muscular and skeletal systems, based in the heels and outer bony edges of both feet, and then the reproductive systems on the triangular inner heels.*

9 *Finally the kidneys, bladder and lymphatic system reflexes are stroked to flush out worked-through thoughts and emotions.*

10 *The session is brought to a close by covering the recipient's feet, then putting the thumbs over the solar plexus reflexes for continued calmness, while quietly asking them to take three deep breaths to return from their deeply relaxed state.*

23

A summary of the massage

In this chapter you will learn:
- *the overall sequence*
- *the general effects of the foot massage*
- *about reflexology's role in the future.*

The overall sequence

The following is to assist you in understanding why the feet are massaged in a particular sequence and to serve as a quick reference.

WARM-UP

Always begin with a general massage, known as the warm-up (steps 3–11). These caressing movements reassure the recipient that it's okay to relax, while creating a trusting relationship between the two of you. It's also an ideal opportunity to get a feel for innermost needs, via their feet.

SORTING OUT THE MIND

The brain and sensory reflexes (steps 12–21) are always massaged first, since the whole body is completely dependent upon the state of mind. The soothing movements can either calm or stimulate the nerves; balance the intellect and intuition; soothe or excite the emotions; pacify or heighten the senses and make sure that the nervous system is constantly aware of everything that's going on, inside and outside the body, so that it can react appropriately.

OPEN AVENUES OF EXPRESSION

With the mind sorted out, the nerves are happy to return to their natural state, helped along by the welcome massage of the spinal reflexes (steps 29–37). This either placates or excites the nerves, while, at the same time, relaxes or strengthens the muscles. It also eases overall tension, improves circulation and augments the natural functioning of all the major organs.

FOR GREATER INNER STRENGTH

The head relies on the neck and throat for a fair exchange of vital life force energies, the clarity of which is influenced by the lymphatic system. Although this system infiltrates the whole body, some areas have a concentration of lymphatic vessels and nodes, which is why there are extra lymph reflexes either sides of the toe necks (steps 22–28). Milking these well goes a long way towards relieving neck and throat tension, opening up the avenues of expression and facilitating the exchange of vital life forces.

CREATE INNER HARMONY

The well-positioned endocrine glands are minuscule members of the body that rely on the blood to transport their hormones to the target glands. The endocrine system responds exceptionally well to reflexology because not only are the glands themselves massaged (steps 38–45), one by one, but also the blood flow is enhanced and the target cells made more receptive to taking in the hormones and putting them to good use. Reflexology balances mind, body and soul, for complete inner harmony and overall wellbeing.

MAKE IT EASIER TO BREATHE

Massaging the balls of the feet (steps 46–50) soothes the respiratory and cardiac systems, making it much easier to breathe.

This, in turn, stabilizes and comforts the heart and regulates the blood flow. Self-esteem and self-worth are boosted and the true spirit has a chance to shine through.

HELP FOOD ON ITS WAY

Stroking and stimulating the sole insteps has a direct effect on the digestive tract (steps 51–75), facilitating the taking in and digesting of all life events. Reflexology nourishes the mind, body and soul and ensures a full appreciation of everything and everybody, which is ideal when it comes to forming and maintaining fulfilling relationships. Massaging the lower halves of both sole insteps also influences the upper parts of the urinary tract, as well as the reproductive and excretory systems, helping to get things moving! This makes the recipient feel completely re-energized and rejuvenated.

BACK TO THE ROOTS

The skeletal and muscular systems, as well as the lower parts of the excretory and reproductive systems, are represented on the heels. Kneading these reflexes (steps 76–93) relaxes the whole body, encouraging the release of worked-through thoughts and emotions. It's the full and active participation in all of life's circumstances that fills the whole persona with renewed energy. This, in turn, revitalizes mind, body and soul, ensuring greater security and happiness within.

FOR THE NEXT LEG

The reflexology session is always completed with a gentle, but invigorating, overall massage (steps 94–103). Now that the feet and body are so at ease, they can be stretched beyond self-imposed limits, which then helps in having a broader outlook and a more affable and flexible approach to life.

The cycles of life defy a linear approach to life.

Reflexology today and in the future

Reflexology was valued as a healing medium for many centuries, but became less popular during the scientific revolution around 300 years ago. It, like many other concepts that link mind, body and soul, was soon dismissed as being unscientific. The body then became treated as some kind of sophisticated machine that could only be serviced and maintained by highly trained, specialized personnel. Consequently many lost touch with their true selves, as well as with their connection to the universe. It became inevitable that 'dis-ease' and unrest would become increasingly widespread. The resultant panic and hysteria worldwide has caused an unhealthy obsession with materialism, frequently leading to intense boredom, extreme emptiness and utter frustration, all of which impoverish the mind, exhaust the body and depress the soul.

There are masses of souls that are literally starved and deprived of the deeper meaning of life, which cannot be found or proven through scientific research: it just is. This is where reflexology can be of assistance. Proof that it, along with all the other natural remedies, is effective, is through the ongoing wellbeing of those who receive it.

Fortunately, there is a renewed interest in these ancient healing practices, now that it's realized that solutions are not confined to the physical world alone. Although many people turn to reflexology as a last resort, when all else has failed, they are constantly astounded at its efficiency. They soon realize that inner peace and harmony are possible, even in these distressing times of violence, confusion and fear.

With more and more people taking responsibility for their health and wellbeing, not only can they heal themselves but, in so doing, play a vital role in healing the planet. Reflexology has a huge role to play in the future, which it is more than capable of doing, by helping individuals to get better at being themselves, as they improve every step of the way.

There is inside you, all of the potential that you wish to be,

All the energy to do whatever you would like to do,

If you imagine yourself as you would like to be, doing what you wish to do,

And every day take a step towards your dream,

Although at times it may seem impossible to hold onto that dream,

One day you shall awake to find that you are the person that you dreamed of,

Doing what you wish to do, simply because you had the courage

To believe in your potential and hold onto your dream!

10 THINGS TO REMEMBER

1 *The warm-up reassures the recipient, making it easier for them to relax.*

2 *The brain and sensory reflexes are balanced first to calm the nerves and, in so doing, pacify the body, so that it's more receptive to being re-energized.*

3 *Massaging the spinal reflexes enhances inner strength and helps in dissipating past weaknesses.*

4 *With the toe necks being so well connected to the lymphatic system, milking these areas eases neck and throat tension, removes any emotional blockages and opens up the avenues of expression.*

5 *Each pair of endocrine gland reflexes is massaged, starting with the pituitary gland reflexes in the big toes, to create overall peace and inner harmony.*

6 *The balls of the feet are then stimulated, opening up the chest and making it easier to breathe, while caressing the heart reflexes encourages the free flow of blood throughout, boosting self-esteem and self-worth.*

7 *The digestive reflexes are followed the whole way through, from the mouth reflexes, on the big toes, to the anus reflexes, on the insides of the heels, to assist in coping with all that is going on and energizing the whole.*

8 *Massaging the heels, which contain the skeletal, muscular, excretory and reproductive system reflexes, provides the strength and flexibility to release toxic thoughts and noxious emotions, making way for new beginnings, so that there is constant progress.*

9   *The reflexology session finishes with an overall massage of both feet, assimilating the energies and broadening the outlook on life.*

10 *Reflexology encourages ongoing health by honouring the authentic self so that each soul can fully recognize and utilize its potential.*

Taking it further

The author, Chris Stormer, is a world acclaimed authority on reflexology and is affectionately known worldwide as the 'universal foot lady'. Her previous books are enjoyed by those with a general interest in this fascinating form of healing; they are also used as text and handbooks in training establishments throughout the world. Furthermore, there is a comprehensive range of charts, DVDs, videos and audio tapes available which can be viewed on www.alwaysb.com.

REFLEXOLOGY BOOKS

Refer to 'Larkin's Reflexology Book list' – the most comprehensive list of reflexology books: http://www.anthonylarkin.com/book-list/

The Language of the Feet, also written by Chris Stormer, provides some fascinating insights, as well as some deeper understanding, of the ever-changing characteristics of the feet. With life being constantly on the move, and needs constantly changing, this book makes it so much easier to tune into individual needs since they can differ greatly from massage to massage!

REFLEXOLOGY PUBLICATION

Reflexology World Magazine
PO Box A107
Arncliffe, NSW 2205
reflexologyworld@yahoo.com.au

REFLEXOLOGY CONTACTS

The author
Chris Stormer
+27 (0) 11 803 1604
+27 (0) 82 855 4255
inspired@worldonline.co.za
www.alwaysb.com

Free website for all natural health practitioners
www.reflexologyinrio.com
www.universallyrio.com

SPECIALIZED REFLEXOLOGY

AURA-SOMA® Colour reflexology – New Zealand
Janice Hill
Tel: +64 (0) 6 357 9318
janice.hill@xtra.co.nz
www.colourconnections.co.nz

Colour reflexology – United Kingdom
Pauline Wills
Tel/fax: +44 (0) 20 8204 7672
info@oracleschoolofcolour.com
www.oracleschoolofcolour.com

REFLEXOLOGY WORKSHOPS AND INFORMATION

For Universal Reflexology and language of the feet workshops and seminars
Sally Teixeira
+55 (0) 21 2522 1341
+44 (0) 7941 646 498
sally@reflexologyinrio.com
www.reflexologyinrio.com
www.universallyrio.com

OK in HEALTH website
www.OKinHealth.com
Canada, USA, UK, Ireland

REFLEXOLOGY ASSOCIATIONS

USA

Reflexology Association of
America
www.reflexology-usa.org/

Please visit this website for a
full listing of US associations,
state by state.

California
Reflexology Association of
California
www.reflexology-ca.org

New York
New York State Reflexology
Association
www.nysraweb.org/

AUSTRALIA

Reflexology Association of
Australia
www.reflexology.org.au/

Melbourne
Australian School of
Reflexology and Relaxation
+61 (0) 3 9898 1890
info@asrr.com.au
www.asrr.com.au

The Australian School of
Reflexology
Tel: +61 (0) 2 4976 3881
Fax: +61 (0) 2 4976 3880
www.reflexologyaustralia.com

CANADA

Reflexology Association of Canada
www.reflexolog.org

NEW ZEALAND

Reflexology New Zealand
www.reflexology.org.nz

SOUTH AFRICA

The South African Reflexology Society
P.O. Box 15070
Panorama 7506
South Africa
www.sareflexology.org.za

SOUTH AMERICA

Rio de Janeiro
Sally Teixeira
Tel: +55 (0) 21 2522 1341
Fax: +55 (0) 21 3627 1341
Rio mobile:
+55 (0) 21 8218 0883
Worldwide mobile:
+44 (0) 7941 646498
sally@reflexologyinrio.com
www.reflexologyinrio.com
www.universallyrio.com

UNITED KINGDOM

Association of Reflexologists
+44 (0) 1823 351 010
info@aor.org.uk
www.aor.org.uk

British Reflexology Association
Nicola Hall
+44 (0) 1886 821207
bra@britreflex.co.uk
www.britreflex.co.uk

ENGLAND

Norfolk
Pathways School of Reflexology
+44 (0) 1603 503 794
www.pathwaysreflexology.co.uk

IRELAND

The National Register of
Reflexologists
http://www.nationalreflexology.ie

The European Institute of
Classical Reflexology
Anthony Larkin
Tel: +353 51 422209
footman@eircom.net

SCOTLAND

Edinburgh
Association of Reflexologists
www.reflexology-uk.net/

End of chapter answers

CHAPTER 1

1 *Reflexology assists in re-establishing the health of mind, body and soul through the firm but gentle massage of feet, alerting latent healing abilities within the mind and body for greater peace and harmony throughout.*

2 *The relaxation aspect of reflexology is important since it is only when the mind and body are truly relaxed and at ease that they can regain and retain excellent health.*

3 *Reflexology is so effective because it effectively clears the whole body of impure thoughts and toxic emotions, thereby re-establishing physical, mental, emotional and spiritual equilibrium.*

4 *When a gland or organ is hyperactive, massaging the feet calms it, whereas hypoactive glands and organs are stimulated.*

5 *There are many ongoing benefits of reflexology because it keeps mind, body and soul in tip-top condition, provided there are regular top-ups.*

6 *No academic prerequisites are required when it comes to learning reflexology and although medical knowledge is useful, it is not essential.*

7 *A reflexology session generally lasts an hour.*

8 *Wearing footwear reduces the feet's innate sensitivity, due to the barrier that occurs between the feet and the undulating surfaces of the ground.*

9 *Feet symbolically represent the journey of the soul. According to Greek legend, any lameness was considered a weakness of the spirit; the Ancient Egyptians believed the soles kept the soul safe inside the body; while witches claimed to absorb their mystical powers from the earth through their feet, which is why they were immediately lifted from the ground when found guilty of practising witchcraft. In most societies feet have been revered or feared at some time.*

10 *When a person is uptight and tense the feet become taut and rigid, limiting their movement and making them more susceptible to problems.*

CHAPTER 2

1 *When orthodox medicine and reflexology are used hand in hand the healing process is accelerated.*

2 *Hippocrates, the acknowledged Father of Medicine, stated that the physical body mirrors the emotions, which, in turn, determine the disposition of the mind.*

3 *The body dislikes a lot of inner conflict, as well as emotional turmoil, or a huge issue being made out of something relatively trivial, so it tends to 'play up'.*

4 *Reflexology can't realign shattered or broken bones but it can create the ideal environment for healing to take place.*

5 *After surgery, reflexology helps to reduce any swellings and inner tension, as well as ease pain and discomfort.*

6 *Massaging the feet assists in making lifestyle changes that benefit the mind, body and soul.*

7 *'Dis-ease' is outer evidence of inner turmoil that is brought to the surface by current circumstances.*

8 *An individual's mindset is important because the mind and body can be completely thrown off track with the soul's purpose by one unhealthy obsession that is exacerbated by the incredible temptations of modern-day living.*

9 *When other forms of complementary healing are used alongside reflexology, the healing process tends to speed up.*

10 *Reiki is the energetic aspect of reflexology used to shift and balance life force energies, while replenishing those parts that lack vitality.*

CHAPTER 3

1 *Your approach to life determines whether you are emotionally in tune or in conflict with the environment, which then influences your state of mind and the consequential ease or 'dis-ease' of your body.*

2 *Uneasiness can be the end product of a long list of complaints and ongoing criticism, which highlight the internal discomfort of trying to live up to the expectations of others.*

3 *A build-up of resentment in the body invariably gets in the way by causing excessive anxiety and unbearable tension.*

4 *The abuse of substances has become so widespread because of the tendency to overreact to situations and due to feeling hopeless and helpless.*

5 *The type of symptoms experienced is determined by an individual's reaction to a disturbing memory or inhibiting belief.*

6 *The blood pressure can be detrimentally affected by constantly trying to avoid emotional conflict, since this puts pressure on the physical body, raising the blood pressure and causing hypertension, whereas overwhelming childhood sadness tends to lower the blood pressure.*

7 *Heaviness in the body and feet is caused by heavy thoughts and overwhelming emotions.*

8 *A craving for material possessions is often indicative of not feeling 'good enough'.*

9 *The body uses symptoms of distress to signal that all is not well.*

10 *Reflexology can be used as a preventative tool by reviving the body's innate capacity to be resourceful and strong, so that it has the stamina and guts to get through anything and everything.*

CHAPTER 4

1 *Anybody and everybody can derive enormous benefits from reflexology, since it enables each individual to find their own two feet.*

2 *An essential part of giving reflexology is that it should be applied sensitively and gently to avoid unnecessary discomfort.*

3 *Reflexology is a safe form of healing because it is non-invasive.*

4 *Extra caution should be applied when there's a deep vein thrombosis.*

5 *There are many benefits of having reflexology while pregnant, the main one being that, with the mother-to-be's body becoming so relaxed, ensures a constant flow of natural life force energies, plus plenty of room for the unborn baby to grow and develop.*

6 *The parent, as well as (or rather than) the child, should receive reflexology, when a young child is sick, because babies and children are energetically aware of their parents' thoughts and feelings, so much so that their wellbeing is intrinsically linked.*

7   *Reflexology assists teenagers by ensuring that there is the appropriate distribution of hormones, which, in turn, encourages greater trust and honesty within their relationships, helping them to step into adulthood with far greater assurance, improved tolerance and more poise.*

8   *The main thing that gets in the way of good health in so many adults is themselves!*

9   *Seniors can benefit enormously from having their feet massaged since it keeps their mind, body and soul agile and alert, while injecting their whole being with a renewed enthusiasm for life.*

10 *Even when only one family member is receiving reflexology, the whole family benefits because that individual becomes so much more relaxed, reasonable and pleasant to live with!*

CHAPTER 5

1   *The changing characteristics of the feet assist when giving reflexology because they display the root cause of anything that is unsettling.*

2   *By the feet reflecting deeply disturbing issues, long before they manifest in the body, potential problems can be determined and dealt with before causing physical, mental or emotional havoc.*

3   *The soles reflect the condition of the soul through their composure and characteristics.*

4   *The feet become uptight and tense when an individual feels uneasy.*

5   *Feet become drained of their vibrancy when the individual feels off-colour.*

6   *The shape of the feet becomes distorted when an individual feels trapped or in a compromising or disadvantageous position or when they feel temporarily disabled, which tends to torture and contort the mind.*

7   *There are numerous 'foot' expressions; here are but a few: 'a foot at another's neck', 'be on a good footing', 'put a foot wrong', 'don't let the grass grow beneath your feet', 'try not to put your foot in it', 'have your feet on the ground', 'find one's feet', 'follow in another's footsteps', 'foot in the door',*

'foot the bill', 'footloose and fancy free', 'foul of foot', 'get off on the wrong foot', 'have the length of someone's foot', 'itchy feet', 'kick dust from under one's feet', 'land on one's feet', 'one foot in the grave', 'pitter patter of little feet', 'put your foot down', 'set foot on virgin soils', 'stand on your own two feet' and 'swept off your feet'.

8   The journey through life becomes arduous and heavy-going when fear, uncertainty, self-doubt and anxiety get in the way of progress.

9   The alpha state of consciousness is experienced when drifting off into the most exquisite and deeply relaxing state of awareness; it's a tranquility frequently enjoyed between wakefulness and sleep.

10 When it comes to getting better, everybody has the choice to be the victim of circumstances or the victor.

CHAPTER 6

1   There are many different foot charts, with varying reflex positions, because knowledge of reflexology has been handed down for so many thousands of years, from generation to generation, that the interpretation of the reflexes has fluctuated.

2   A primary reflex provides direct access to a reflex, whereas a secondary or indirect reflex is usually on the opposite side of the foot, providing an alternative or indirect approach to the reflex.

3   The body is reflected onto both feet, in miniature, with the front being mirrored onto the soles and the back onto the tops. The right side of the body is reflected onto the right foot and the left side of the body is mirrored onto the left foot.

4   Reflexes that rebound throughout both feet are the nerves, blood and lymph vessels, plus bones and muscles.

5   The upper surfaces of the feet represent the back of the body.

6   When a bone is crushed or shattered, its reflex has a splintered or gritty feel about it.

7   The parts of the feet that reflect the front of the body are the soles.

8 *The arms and legs are reflected onto the outer edges of both feet, although the legs are also reflected, in a seated position, onto the soles of both feet.*

9 *The root cause of back problems is unresolved issues, disturbing memories and unreasonable beliefs that linger in the background.*

10 *The 'inner edges' refers to all the medial aspects of the feet and toes while the 'outer edges' are all the lateral surfaces of the feet.*

CHAPTER 7

1 *Touch is important since it eases distress, pacifies emotions, reassures the soul, induces confidence, creates trust and increases acceptance of oneself and others.*

2 *You should approach reflexology in your own unique way because you are an individual and your approach to reflexology is unique; nobody can touch another soul quite like you.*

3 *It's best to touch feet with supreme sensitivity, the purest of intent and complete acceptance.*

4 *Tuning into the recipient's energy provides insight as to how to intuitively touch them, be it firm, medium or light.*

5 *The amount of pressure applied when massaging feet should vary according to the recipient's ever-changing needs.*

6 *The need to be lovingly touched increases during times of illness, distress or insecurity.*

7 *Using all digits enhances the treatment because each digit has its own unique energy, which alters the vibration, as well as the effect of the massage; this introduces a far greater range of healing possibilities.*

8 *The reflexes that require special attention are those of the brain, spine, solar plexus and endocrine system, as well as congested, swollen areas or parts that lack energy and vibrancy.*

9 *The thumbs re-establish trust, creating a much-needed balance between the intellect and intuition; the index fingers highlight innermost feelings; the middle fingers activate innovative*

ideas; the ring fingers encourage the communication of new concepts; while the little fingers bring to the fore individuality and uniqueness.

10   You should resist the temptation to take credit for the healing so that you don't lose confidence when, from time to time, the recipient chooses not to get better.

CHAPTER 8

1   The natural state of healthy feet is vibrant and pliable.

2   The skin on the feet hardens and thickens whenever the going gets tough. Calluses and corns highlight areas of extreme susceptibility, conceal true feelings or may even be covering up perceived inadequacies.

3   Feet become flaccid when giving in too easily under pressure or when lacking the inner strength and substance to keep going.

4   The colours on the feet tend to vary so much because they mirror shifts in overriding moods and uppermost emotions.

5   The various colours on the feet are: white, which indicates being absolutely drained, tired and exhausted, or is a sign of divine guidance and enlightenment; black or blue from momentarily being in the dark, or desperately needing an expressive outlet, or when really hurt and emotionally battered; green comes from extreme envy or a profound need to just be; yellow indicates exceptional annoyance, or a jaundiced view of life, or even being overly conscientious; orange reveals mixed emotions about conveying something important, or else feeling really fed up and confused; red is usually a sign of heated emotions, intense rage, extreme frustration, total embarrassment or surfacing passion; and, brown occurs when 'browned off', or when there's a need to feel more grounded, or the feet may just be dirty!

6   The right foot tends to reflect past issues.

7   The angle of the feet signifies an individual's perceived position, bearing and progress in life.

8   When walking the feet should point directly ahead and be parallel.

9   *While standing, the gap between the feet implies the degree of openness to what's going on, as well as the scope of interest.*

10 *When the recipient is lying flat on their back, the feet should remain upright but supple.*

CHAPTER 9

1   *The brain reflexes can be found on all the toe pads.*

2   *The brain reflexes reveal the content or discontent of the mind.*

3   *The face is mirrored onto the toe pads to reveal how well life is being 'faced'.*

4   *The aspects of the mind that each pair of toes reflects is as follows: the 'intellectual' big toes resonate to innermost beliefs, as well as intuitive and spiritual choices; the 'emotional' second toes are full of opinions about oneself and others; the 'enterprising' third toes have a wealth of bright ideas about what to do or not do; the 'chatty' fourth toes reveal a host of views related to personal relationships, as well as the way in which to communicate; and the little 'family' toes disclose the amount of inner security with one's own way of thinking.*

5   *The massage should be focused on the tips of the toes to soothe extreme sensitivity, ease intense irritability and increase the level of tolerance, especially when there's sinus congestion, allergies or fits of rage. Additional attention is given to these reflexes for baldness, depression, dizziness, vertigo, fainting, headaches, insomnia and any type of nervousness.*

6   *The forehead and midbrain reflexes display the nature of deep thoughts, as well as the impressions gained in life.*

7   *The toenails represent the skull and the back of the head.*

8   *A corn can develop when personal ideas and beliefs are being threatened or to prevent personal ideas from being 'stamped out' or to avoid 'getting it in the neck' or 'turning a deaf ear'.*

9   *Social constraints and detrimental beliefs put a huge amount of pressure on the mind.*

10 *Thoughts alter the natural state. Set ideas, an unbending attitude, an obdurate approach to life, uncertainty and insecurity, all tend to make the toes stiffen and change their stance.*

CHAPTER 10

1 *The shape of the toes reveals how ideas take shape, which then influences the shape of things to come.*
2 *The toe pads change shape whenever thoughts form in a particular way or when there's a complete change of mind.*
3 *The words you use to describe your toes provide invaluable insight into your innermost thoughts.*
4 *The size of your toes indicates how you size up your own ideas, influencing what you think of other ways of thinking.*
5 *Toe pads provide useful insight into the workings of a person's mind and reveal whether or not they are facing the world with their incredible ideas.*
6 *The condition of the skin on your feet, especially on the toes, reveal the impact of conditioned belief systems, as well as deeply ingrained memories regarding 'kin'.*
7 *Anything you dislike about the skin on your feet is drawing your attention to areas of concern, particularly amongst those family members who tend to 'get under the skin'.*
8 *If there is hard skin, especially on the toes, it could mean that you find it hard to think in the same way as others, or you are having difficulty in being yourself.*
9 *Blisters can occur when there's a conflict of interests.*
10 *Ideally the feet should be massaged at least once a day.*

CHAPTER 11

1 *Back and neck tension can be immediately eased by massaging the corresponding reflexes on the feet.*
2 *The spinal reflexes are massaged well to renew sensitivity and reinforce ongoing support and backing.*
3 *The spinal reflexes are stimulated when the nerves are insensitive or non-reactive; they are soothed when there's a high level of irritability, too much sensitively or extreme intolerance.*
4 *The arches of the feet represent an individual's ability to stay 'in step' or 'out of step' with the general way of thinking; they also reveal the inner strength to go against the 'norm'.*

5 *The arches can fall flat and collapse when there's immense emotional strain, making it impossible to 'stand up for oneself'; meanwhile they become over-extended to provide additional support during exceptionally challenging periods, or when 'bending over backwards' to please others.*

6 *When under strain, the nervous impulses tend to become distorted or traumatized, with the smallest irritation sending them off at a tangent, often resulting in a 'bad' reaction.*

7 *Detrimental thoughts upset the body, until they eventually 'get on the nerves', causing tension in both the body and the feet.*

8 *The hand reflexes are the soft mounds, in front of the outer ankle bones, on the tops of both feet; they reflect the handling of life and ability to deal with ongoing events.*

9 *No, it's not essential to find the foot reflexes because they are so tiny and the feet are already receiving a full massage.*

10 *Massaging the toes and arches has far-reaching effects because they are linked to the nervous system and, therefore, every cell is influenced to some degree or other.*

CHAPTER 12

1 *Your description of your big toes will help you to understand whether you are really on track with your soul mission and, if not, why.*

2 *Massaging the big toes contributes to the wellbeing of the whole body by providing space in which to think and connecting the mind to the creative source.*

3 *The natural state of the big toes and toe necks is upright and supple.*

4 *The need to be overly controlling arises from a deep fear of not being in control.*

5 *The big toes require extra attention, when being massaged, for all nervous, endocrine and sensory disorders.*

6 *The role of the endocrine system is to maintain a harmonious inner environment, which then sets the tone for the whole body.*

7 *Reflexology balances the endocrine system by ensuring a healthy hormonal production, also by ensuring that the hormones are fairly distributed through vibrant blood vessels*

and finally by making sure the target cells make the best use of the hormones.

8   The sensory system contributes to overall health by creating awareness of what's going on internally and externally so that there are meaningful and beneficial interactions.

9   The various senses of the body are linked to specific toes. The inner sense is linked to the big toes and toe necks; sight is related to the second toes; the sense of smell and detection of sound are allied to third toes; taste is connected to the fourth toes; and touch is sensed by the little toes.

10   Reflexology is extremely effective, when it comes to massaging the sensory reflexes, because it puts things into perspective; this is especially useful when the perception of stimuli is distorted.

CHAPTER 13

1   The reflexes found on the toe necks are those of the neck and throat. Their condition is affected by the ability to express personal concepts and ideas.

2   The cervical bone reflexes are along the inner edges of both big toe necks.

3   When true self-expression is stifled, it can lead to anger, guilt, stubbornness or a fear of 'speaking up', which effectively chokes and throttles individuality.

4   The feet tend to cramp when there's a gripping fear or concern about having 'one's style cramped'.

5   The major body system connected to expressive areas is the lymphatic system.

6   Should you have any markings, lumps and swellings on your toe necks, it could either be a collection of unexpressed emotion, if on the inner edges, or a post-nasal drip, from not being able to cry openly, if on the outer edges.

7   The thyroid gland reflexes reflect an innate desire to 'spread one's wings and fly', free of any constraints or restrictions. Massaging these reflexes creates more space for self-expression, while boosting confidence and re-energizing the whole body.

8 *Massaging hyperactive glands calms them down, whereas massaging hypoactive glands stimulates them.*

9 *If there are a lot of 'shoulds' or 'shouldn'ts' in your life, you will find their energy accumulating in your shoulders, which is then reflected onto the strips immediately beneath the toe necks.*

10 *The wrist reflexes are immediately under the outer ankle bones, while the ankle reflexes are just below them. Massaging the tiny wrist reflexes creates greater flexibility when handling life's situations, while massaging the miniscule ankle reflexes assists in adapting to the ups and downs that are encountered on the journey through life.*

CHAPTER 14

1 *The word 'emotion' can be derived from 'energy in motion', with the 'energy' being 'thoughts' and the 'motion' their movement through the body. The motion of thoughts arouses deep memories and unlocks suppressed feelings.*

2 *The major systems and organs connected to feelings are the respiratory system, the heart and circulatory system, as well as the eyes, index fingers, bottom halves of the lower arms and shins, breasts and chest.*

3 *The eye reflexes are on the central mounds of all toe pads. Their importance comes from being the windows to the soul.*

4 *Intuition is the 'inner tutor' or 'gut feel' that provides a 'deep knowing'. To enhance this innate gift, let your imagination run wild.*

5 *The reflexes mirrored onto the balls of the feet are the chest, breasts, ribcage, lungs, thymus gland, upper arm, airways and oesophagus.*

6 *The changing colours on the feet mirror changes of emotion.*

7 *The chest and breast reflexes reveal the impact that feelings have on personal wellbeing.*

8 *Massaging the thymus gland reflexes reconnects the individual with their true spirit, making them proud to be unique.*

9 *The solar plexus reflexes are believed to be the most powerful reflexes on the feet because massaging them induces instant calm that spreads throughout the whole.*

10 *The heart reflexes are on the inside edges, where the balls of the feet and the insteps meet, with the larger reflex being on the left foot. The circulation of blood is affected by the acceptance or non-acceptance of oneself and others.*

CHAPTER 15

1 *The condition of the third toes is influenced by thoughts of what to do or not do.*

2 *The third toes are energetically connected to the middle fingers, the cheeks, ears, nose, upper abdomen, as well as the top halves of the lower arms and lower shins.*

3 *The nose reflexes are halfway along the inner edges of each toe, the ear reflexes are midway along the outer edges of the toes, while the cheek reflexes are the small bulges, just off the centre of all the toes. The nose plays up when irritated; the ears by what is said or not said; and the cheeks from being considered to be impudent.*

4 *The type of inputs that detrimentally affect the digestive tract are the extremes of emotions and negative thoughts.*

5 *The liver and gall bladder reflexes change their appearance and become distended with anger, resentment or bitterness; whereas they sink from utter exasperation, especially when pressured into meeting ludicrous social and family expectations.*

6 *Nasty thoughts and noxious emotions are toxic to the body.*

7 *Massaging the pancreatic and splenic reflexes puts any unhappiness that causes diabetes into perspective while, at the same time, easing any form of obsessive behavior. As for hypoglycaemia, reflexology restores the enthusiasm for life.*

8 *No, the right and left adrenal gland reflexes are not in the same position. Although they are both immediately beneath the solar plexus reflexes, the right reflex is slightly lower and a little more central than the left. They provide incredible courage and resourcefulness for unique and innovative ideas to be put into practice, regardless of any initial disapproval, adversity or criticism.*

9   *The stomach is easily upset by unexpected events, ongoing inactivity, deep dread, extreme concern or fear of taking on something new or unusual; the cardiac sphincter is affected by overwhelming emotions, while the pyloric sphincter is influenced by the ability to process all that has been taken in, depending on what happened previously. Massaging these reflexes makes stomaching life's events more manageable, restores faith in personal capabilities and provides the reassurance to move on despite what happened in the past.*

10 *The middle back reflexes are reflected around the upper halves of both insteps. Their appearance is influenced by the amount and type of backing and support given to oneself and others.*

CHAPTER 16

1 *The thoughts that the fourth toes and lower insteps pick up on are all about communications and relationships.*

2 *The fourth toes are energetically linked to the mouth, ring fingers, bottom halves of the upper arms and thighs, as well as the lower abdomen.*

3 *The element that is affected by what is going on within relationships is water.*

4 *The colour that reveals the amount of joy and happiness being derived from life is orange.*

5 *The mouth reflexes are three-quarters of the way down the inner edges of all the toes; the small intestine reflexes occupy the bulk of the lower halves of both sole insteps; the ileo-caecal valve reflex is on the outer lower corner of the right sole instep and just below it is the appendix reflex. The mouth's functioning is affected by the energy of words, spoken and unspoken; the small intestines by the absorption of new life force energies; the ileo-caecal valve by the onward movement of anything that is no longer required in the body and the appendix by dead-end relationships.*

6 *The female reproductive organs that are related to the fourth toes are the ovaries, with reflexes in the outer lower corner of both sole insteps, and the fallopian tubes and their fingers, with reflexes stretching across the soles, along or near the base of the fleshy sole instep, just above the heels.*

7   The role of the kidneys is to do the initial processing of worked-through thoughts and obsolete emotions that need to be released. Their reflexes are tiny, kidney-shaped vertical mounds, on the lower sole instep areas, immediately beneath the adrenal gland reflexes, with the right reflex being slightly lower and a fraction further in towards the centre of the right foot, than on the left.

8   The upper arm reflexes are significant because they reveal the willingness to reach out and welcome new beginnings, according to the belief in oneself.

9   The lumbar vertebrae reflexes are connected to the fourth toes because of their ability to provide support and backup within personal relationships.

10 Reflexology assists digestion by calming down the whole process, making it much easier to deal with daily events and cope with everything on one's plate.

CHAPTER 17

1   The height and stature of the little toes signify the effect of family and social belief systems on an individual's status at home and, subsequently, their standing in society.

2   There are four major bodily systems connected to the little toes, which include the excretory, reproductive, skeletal and muscular systems.

3   The element that has the greatest influence on the little toes is earth, while the colour they resonate to the best is a deep passionate red.

4   The jaw reflexes are situated along the underneath edges of all the toe pads.

5   Your likes and dislikes of your heels highlight your satisfaction or dissatisfaction about the progress you have made or are making. To change their characteristics and improve them, get rid of any self-imposed limitations that hold back your mind and body.

6   The strength of the bones signifies inner substance and the resourcefulness to deal with life's 'ups and downs', while muscles provide the body and feet with the flexibility

to adapt and expand to ensure personal growth and development.

7   The pelvic bone reflexes occupy the bulk of the heel pads; the hip reflexes are on the outer ankle bones: the buttock reflexes are the rounded aspect of the heels, below the outer ankle bones; the arc-shaped rectum reflexes are on the inner surfaces of both heels and the anus reflexes are small palpable indentations, midway between the inner ankle bones and tips of the inside heels.

8   The bladder reflexes should appear as fleshy mounds.

9   The lower reproductive organ and gland reflexes situated on the inside of both ankles are the uterus and vagina on females, and the testes and penis on men.

10   The lower back reflexes change and become distended when reaching out for more support and financial backing, whereas they sink due to insufficient funds or when there's a drain on personal resources.

CHAPTER 18

1   Reflexology assists the father-to-be, before pregnancy, to produce stronger, healthier sperm and also provides him with the inner strength and confidence to give support throughout; for the mother-to-be, it helps to create a far more conducive womb environment, boosts her resources, increases her awareness of her role as a mother and enhances her intuitive abilities, all of which makes the unborn baby feel most welcome.

2   The feet being regularly massaged throughout the pregnancy reassures the mother-to-be that she can and will cope and reduces the risk of complications. This, in turn, ensures a good supply of vital life force energies to the womb for the healthy development of the baby.

3   With the womb being so receptive and providing such a loving space, the unborn baby is able to grow and develop to its full potential.

4   Reflexology encourages the father-to-be to become more supportive and understanding, which helps him feel more competent.

5 Around six to eight weeks after conception, the embryo reflexes can be seen on one of the uterine reflexes, on the inside edge; if only on one foot it's likely to be just one baby, but if on both feet it could be twins.

6 Should the baby be in a breech position, rotating the mother-to-be's little toes has been known to encourage the unborn baby to turn.

7 When the father-to-be massages his partner's feet during childbirth, it not only calms, relaxes and reassures both of them but keeps the expectant father well occupied, and makes him feel useful.

8 When the mother-to-be is ready to give birth, it's possible that her big toes will pull back, while all her other toes will extend forwards.

9 It's really beneficial for all family members to have their feet massaged after the baby is born because everybody is far more relaxed and stays much calmer, which is exceptionally reassuring for the baby.

10 You should feel really confident about massaging a pregnant woman's feet, knowing that the benefits of reflexology are invaluable when it comes to falling pregnant, carrying the baby, as well as during and after the birth.

CHAPTER 19

1 There are four basic movements in reflexology.

2 The rotation technique creates an energetic link with the universe; the caterpillar movement improves the physique; the stroking or milking method soothes emotions and the feathering or healing caress reacquaints the recipient with their authentic self.

3 The approach should vary, when massaging the feet, so that the technique can be adjusted to meet the ever-changing needs of the individual.

4 Knowing exactly how much pressure to apply is an intuitive process that cannot be taught. It's a matter of feeling your way!

5 It's best to practise the technique on yourself to gain the confidence to do it on others.

6   *The energy channels of the mind, body and soul open when
    the digits are placed onto a reflex, slight pressure is applied for
    a while and then slowly released. Otherwise the digit can be
    gently gyrated for as long as necessary.*

7   *Tension, pain and distress are eased by reflexology through the
    caterpillar movement, which involves 'walking' the thumbs.*

8   *The most soothing technique is the stroking or milking
    movement.*

9   *The soul is reconnected with its true spirit by the feathering
    or healing caress.*

10 *It's important to get to know yourself better because, by
    understanding your authentic self, you can create the most
    enriching and enlightening experience for yourself on earth.*

CHAPTER 20

1   *Everybody's experience is so different because everybody is
    an individual, with their own unique experience and personal
    beliefs.*

2   *No, since it depends on their willingness to release past
    experiences and outdated beliefs.*

3   *Some of the more common responses to reflexology are heat
    loss, extreme tenderness over certain reflexes, a sinking or
    floating sensation, twitching, jerking, snoring and seeing a
    variety of colours.*

4   *Some of the less likely reactions include plucking hand
    movements, out-of-body experiences, recall of previous life
    situations, and singing out loud, to mention but a few.*

5   *It's important to explain possible side-effects to the recipient
    since they need to realize that, no matter what, reflexology
    works with, and not against, the manifestations of illness,
    for ultimate healing to take place.*

6   *Most people feel absolutely fantastic after a reflexology
    session; full of energy with a huge sense of relief!*

7   *Some of the ways in which the body cleanses itself of toxic
    thoughts and noxious emotions are through headaches, high
    temperatures, increased perspiration, runny eyes, a cold
    or runny nose, skin rashes or eruptions, a virulent vaginal*

discharge in women, increased urination, frequent, easier defecation, temporary diarrhoea and a vivid recall of dreams.

8 Drinking plenty of purified water helps to flush away the past after a reflexology massage.

9 If an unusual or frightening reaction happens, just remain calm; immediately place your thumbs or middle fingers onto the solar plexus reflexes and allow yourself to be intuitively guided into knowing what to do next. Remind yourself that reflexology is a non-invasive, natural therapy, so only dormant issues, already resident in the body, can be brought to the fore.

10 A further treatment, after an excessive reaction to reflexology, is best within a day or two, to bring mind, body and soul back into balance.

CHAPTER 21

1 The best way to treat emotional wounds is to lovingly caress and stroke their corresponding reflexes on the feet.

2 The two most essential tools when it comes to giving reflexology are the hands and the heart.

3 The most congenial and tranquil healing environment can be created by using a dimmer switch and/or a softly flickering candle, by burning aromatherapy oils or an incense stick, by playing soothing music in the background, by placing a 'Do not disturb' notice on the door and by activating a telephone answering machine or service.

4 A simple and clear explanation should be given to the recipient before starting the treatment because it helps to reassure and relax them.

5 Once those on prescribed medication have advised their specialist of their intention to have reflexology, they should ideally receive their treatments an hour before the next dosage is due.

6 To make the recipient feel comfortable, soak their feet in warm or cool water. Once their feet are dry, invite them to lie flat on a bed or couch, placing one pillow beneath their head and another one or two pillows under their knees and lower legs, to make sure that their spine is straight and flat. Finally, cover their body with a light sheet or warm blanket.

7   If you prefer to use powder, it's likely that you like to feel
    what's going on at a deeper level, whereas a preference for oil
    could be because you enjoy flowing movements.

8   Conversation during the treatment is discouraged, so that
    the recipient can drift off into the tranquil alpha state of
    consciousness and reconnect with their inner self.

9   It's important to understand that it is the recipient who heals
    themselves because they need to be acknowledged and retain
    their personal power.

10 When going from one foot to the other, the right foot should
    ideally be massaged first because it represents the past.

CHAPTER 22

1   Both feet are simultaneously massaged, when giving
    reflexology, to provide an overall balance and to keep the two
    feet energetically connected.

2   The treatment starts at the tips of the toes and gradually
    progresses down the feet because everything begins as a
    thought; then as this thought runs through the body, it
    evokes feelings, which, in turn, get a reaction, that once
    communicated affects an individual's inner security and
    overall wellbeing.

3   The warm-up sequence encourages the recipient to relax and
    provides time to connect and gauge what's going on at a much
    deeper level.

4   The energy channels of the body and soul can be opened and
    re-energized, via the feet, by gently placing the fingertips onto
    the tips of each of the corresponding toes and applying slight
    pressure for a few seconds; then easing off until the fingertips
    are resting or hovering above the toe surfaces.

5   The feet are caressed and stroked all over, between each
    sequence, as a caring way of creating overall harmony, to
    accelerate the healing process and to reassure the recipient.
    It is also a very effective way of warming cold feet.

6   The first and most essential reflexes that need to be focused
    on are those of the nervous system reflexes since the brain
    controls the functioning of the whole body.

7   The sequence always begins with a general massage, known as the 'warm-up'; followed by massaging the nerve, spinal, endocrine and sensory reflexes on all the toes; then the neck and throat reflexes on the toe necks; the respiratory and cardiac reflexes on the balls of the feet; the digestive reflexes on both insteps and finally the skeletal, muscular, reproductive and excretory reflexes on the heels; finishing with a gentle, but invigorating, overall massage, known as the 'finale'.

8   Drawing your own feet on a piece of paper and then drawing in the various reflexes helps enormously in knowing which reflex is where on the feet.

9   The kidneys, bladder and lymphatic reflexes are caressed towards the end of a reflexology treatment to ensure that all worked-through thoughts and emotions are released and eliminated.

10 The reflexology sequence is completed by the massage of the solar plexus reflexes, followed by stroking first the right foot, from top to bottom, and then the left foot. Both feet should then be covered and held, with the recipient being invited to take in three deep breaths, to ground them and to allow them to surface in their own time. A glass of water also brings them back to earth, while further flushing out the old from their systems.

Appendix I

Healing enhanced through the use of oils

The sensuous aspect of aromatherapy oils has a therapeutic effect on mind, body and soul. A mixture of one to three oils, within approximately 30 ml of base oil, rubbed into the feet, at the end of a reflexology session, really enhances its effects. There are six main types of oil:

Uplifting oils	Boost confidence, ease depression and eliminate moodiness. Examples include clary sage, jasmine and grapefruit.
Regulating oils	Relieve anxiety and re-establish equilibrium. Examples include bergamot, frankincense, geranium and rosewood.
Stimulating oils	Strengthen concentration, clear the mind and improve memory. Examples include lemon, peppermint, rosemary and black pepper.
Invigorating oils	Fill the whole being with enthusiasm and interest, thereby strengthening the immune system. Examples include cardamom, juniper, rosemary and lemongrass.
Soothing oils	Increase levels of tolerance, improve sleep patterns and calm the mind. Examples include chamomile, lavender, marjoram and orange blossom.
Aphrodisiac oils	Strengthen relationships and boost self-esteem. Examples are clary sage, patchouli and ylang ylang.

Appendix II

The vibrancy of colours for inner harmony

Visualization of colours during reflexology alters the vibrational tone of the healing energies, which are then absorbed into the body, to fine-tune mind, body and soul, harmonizing them for overall balance. The following guide suggests which colours to visualize but, should another colour come to mind while you are massaging the feet, then visualize that colour instead.

Red	Fifth toes and heels	Provides security, mobility and enthusiasm for ongoing development. 'See red' when things get in the way of one's progress.
Orange	Fourth toes and lower halves of instep	Communicates the joy of feeling secure in one's relationships, making life such a pleasure.
Yellow	Third toes and upper halves of insteps	Provides the passion to instigate ideas and make them a reality.
Green	Second toes and balls of the feet	Harmonizes the internal and external environments, creating space in which to be oneself.
Blue	Toe necks	Clears the way for the exchange of life force energies, closing the gap between the physical and non-physical.
Purple	All toes	By clearing the mind, it provides space in which to think and to find an inner peace and balance by reconnecting with the divine source.

Appendix III

Music to relax the body, mind and soul

There's a huge selection of beautiful music, ideal for playing while giving reflexology. The following are a few suggestions to help you on your way.

Reflexology music	*Universal Reflexology – The Healing Journey* – two discs, with the procedure narrated by Sally Teixeira with specially composed music, compiled by Courtney Ward. *Spirit Song* – A wonderful CD using indigenous instruments that gently stir and release deeply suppressed memories (Courtney Ward).
Dolphin and whale	Particularly beneficial during pregnancy and childbirth, as well as for special needs children and for disturbed, restless souls.
Natural sounds	Such as wind, birdsong, waterfalls and waves. Examples are: *Wilderness* by Tony O'Conner, *Wetland Symphony* by Ducks Unlimited, Canada.
Ethnic music	Using traditional instruments such as drums, didgeridoos, panflutes and so on. Examples include: *Eagle* by Medwin Goodall, *Uluru* by Tony O'Connor.
Electric harp	An example is: *Dream Spiral* by Hilary Stagg.
Others	*Gifts of the Angels* by Steven Halpern *Bushland Dreaming* by Tony O'Connor *Inner Tides* by Ian Cameron Smith.

Appendix IV

Getting on the nerves

	Irritability	Tolerance	Patience	Sensitivity
Too much	Sets the 'nerves on edge'	Complete intolerance or too much acceptance and leniency can manifest as an allergic reaction.	Endurance and persistence that test patience until no more can be taken.	Overly concerned and anxious from becoming too involved, with the tendency to overreact and take umbrage.
Too little	Numbness or paralysis from 'deadening of the nerves' to eliminate the pain of a terrible memory or distressing belief.	The 'disease' to please causes inner antagonism and suppressed ill feelings towards others.	Impatience leads to edginess and agitation.	Appear indifferent, unresponsive, cold or unconcerned to conceal a past upset or deep hurt.

Index

abdominal cavity, *43*
abdominal cramps, *141*
abscesses, *129*
abuse of substances, *18–19*
accidents, *168*
aches, *81*
Achilles tendon, *220–2*
acne, *168*
acupressure, *14*
acupuncture, *14*
addiction, *108, 138*
Addison's disease, *139*
adenoid disorders, *130*
adolescents, *27*
adrenal gland, *44, 139–40, 251*
adults, *27–8*
ageing, *168–9*
AIDS, *114*
air embolisms, *106*
airway, *116*
alcohol/alcoholism, *18, 135*
Alexander Technique, *13*
allergies, *66*
alpha level of consciousness, *36, 200*
Alzheimer's disease, *89–90*
amnesia, *90*
anaemia, *124*
ankles, *10, 45, 100, 217–18*
anorexia, *109*
anus, *44, 175–6, 273*
appendicitis, *155*
appendix, *42, 155, 267–8*

arches, *79–80, 83–4, 239*
arms
    lower, *42, 121, 277*
    upper, *45, 161, 276*
aromatherapy, *13, 209, 331*
arteriosclerosis, *124*
arthritis, *138*
ascending colon, *156, 268*
asphyxiating attacks, *112*
asthma, *112, 245*
attention-deficient children, *26*

babies
    breast feeding, *113*
    in breech position, *188*
    reflexology for, *26, 190*
    see also children
back
    disorders, *43, 45, 78, 79, 162, 182, 188*
    lower, *182–3, 243*
    middle, *129, 144–5, 162, 241–2, 273–4*
    upper, *122, 241*
    see also spine
balance, loss of, *131*
baldness, *65, 66*
balls of the feet, *43, 109–10, 297–8*
bed wetting, *177*
belching, *106, 109*
belief systems, *68–9, 74–5, 166–7*
Bell's palsy, *67*

big toes, *43, 64–5, 84, 87–9, 91*
bladder, *44, 176–7, 286–7*
bleeding, *124, 152*
blindness, *107*
blisters, *75, 153*
blood, *124–5, 188*
body odour, *129*
boils, *135*
bones, *170–1*
    see also skeletal system
bowels, *156–7*
    see also colon
boxed toes, *75*
brain, *44, 63–4, 65–6, 81, 237, 296*
brain tumours, *67*
breast cysts, *113*
breasts, *41, 42, 43, 112–13, 188, 255*
breathing, *111–12, 123, 297–8*
    during session, *214–15, 292*
broken bones, *170*
bronchial spasms, *245*
bruising, *90*
bulimia, *138*
bunions, *114, 121*
burns, *134*
bursitis, *170*
buttocks, *173–4, 280–1*

calluses, *110, 168*
cancer, *108, 109*
candida, *153*
cardiac sphincter, *42, 140–1, 263*
cardiac system, *253–4, 297*
    see also heart
carpal tunnel syndrome, *99*
cataracts, *107*

caterpillar movement, *193, 194–5*
cellulite, *138*
cerebral palsy, *152*
cheeks, *132*
chest, *43*
chest congestion, *112*
childbirth, *189–90*
childhood ailments, *160*
children
    bed wetting, *177*
    reflexology for, *26–7*
    see also babies
chills, *134–5*
cholesterol issues, *125*
cigarettes, *18, 21*
circulation, *124–5*
cold sores, *152*
colds, *130, 135, 203*
colic, *156*
colitis, *156*
colon, *42, 44, 156–7, 268–72*
colour
    feet, *57–8*
    toes, *75*
    visualisation, *332*
colour healing, *13*
coma, *107*
communication, *209–10*
complementary therapies, *13–14*
conception, *186*
conjunctivitis, *107*
consciousness, alpha level, *36, 200*
constipation, *138, 176*
convulsions, *81*
corns, *68*
cramps, *96, 141, 172*

Image credits

Notes